Chemotherapeutic Strategy

Chemotherapeutic Strategy

Proceedings of the Symposium held on June 2-4 1982
at the World Trade Centre, London UK

Edited by

D I EDWARDS

and

D R HISCOCK

Chemotherapy Research Unit
Department of Paramedical Sciences
North East London Polytechnic
London E15 4LZ

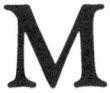

First published 1983 by
Scientific and Medical Division
THE MACMILLAN PRESS LTD.
London and Basingstoke
Companies and representatives throughout the world

ISBN 978-1-349-06542-4   ISBN 978-1-349-06540-0 (eBook)
DOI 10.1007/978-1-349-06540-0

*The organisers of the Symposium and editors of the book are
indebted to the following who provided
sponsorship for the meeting on
Chemotherapeutic Strategy*

Beecham Pharmaceuticals Ltd
Janssen Pharmaceuticals Ltd
The Macmillan Press
May and Baker Ltd
Roche Products Ltd
Roussel Laboratories Ltd
Squibb & Sons Ltd
Upjohn Ltd

Contents

The Contributors

E Cundliffe
Department of Biochemistry
University of Leicester
Adrian Building
University Road
Leicester LE1 7RH, UK

D I Edwards
Chemotherapy Research Unit
Department of Paramedical
   Sciences
North East London Polytechnic
Romford Road
London E15 4LZ, UK

G Gregoriadis
Division of Clinical Sciences
Clinical Research Centre
Watford Road
Harrow
Middlesex HA1 3UJ, UK

S M Hammond
Department of Microbiology
University of Leeds
Leeds LS2 9JT, UK

K Hellmann
Cancer Chemotherapy Department
Imperial Cancer Research Fund
P O Box 123
Lincoln's Inn Fields
London WC2A 3PX, UK

D R Hiscock
Department of Paramedical
   Sciences
North East London Polytechnic
Romford Road
London E15 4LZ, UK

R E Howells
Department of Parasitology
Liverpool School of Tropical
   Medicine
Pembroke Place
Liverpool L3 5QA, UK

S Neidle
Cancer Research Campaign
   Biomolecular Structure
   Research Group
Department of Biophysics
King's College
26-29 Drury Lane
London WC2B 5RL, UK

B A Newton
Medical Research Council Unit
   for Biochemical Parasitology
The Molteno Institute
Downing Street
Cambridge CB2 3EE, UK

S Selwyn
Department of Medical
  Microbiology
Westminster Medical School
Horseferry Road
London SW1P 2AR, UK

J T Smith
The Microbiology Section
Department of Pharmaceutics
The School of Pharmacy
University of London
Brunswick Square
London WC1N 1AX, UK

I J Stratford
Radiobiology Group
Department of Physics
Institute of Cancer Research
Clifton Avenue
Sutton
Surrey SM2 5PX, UK

J P Tollenaere
Department of Theoretical
  Medicinal Chemistry
Janssen Pharmaceutica
B-2340 Beerse, Belgium

P Wardman
Cancer Research Campaign
Gray Laboratory
Mount Vernon Hospital
Northwood
Middlesex HA6 2RN, UK

A T Willis
Public Health Laboratory
Luton and Dunstable Hospital
Lewsey Road
Luton LU4 0DZ, UK

Chemotherapeutic Strategy – An Overview

D I Edwards and D R Hiscock

Department of Paramedical Sciences
North East London Polytechnic
Romford Road, London E15 4LZ, UK

This volume reports the proceedings of a symposium on Chemotherapeutic Strategy held at the World Trade Centre, London in June
1982 and which was organised by the Chemotherapy Research Unit of
North East London Polytechnic. During the Symposium three major
aspects of chemotherapeutic strategy were discussed; the targets
within the susceptible cell (including resistance), problems of the
chemotherapy of infection (including cancer), and lastly, new
approaches to chemotherapeutic strategy which are of current
interest and which may prove of greater value in the future.

The scope of the Symposium was intended to encompass as broad
an area as possible so as to afford the opportunity to stimulate
common ideas and approaches. The use of liposomes in drug targeting
for example may not ultimately prove to be of use in cancer but the
idea has been adopted for other drug delivery systems including
antiprotozoal chemotherapy. Similarly, a knowledge of free radicals
is essential in understanding the action and selective toxicity of
nitroimidazole drugs in anaerobic protozoal and bacterial chemotherapy as well as their enormous potential as radiosensitizers for
the treatment of hypoxic tumours in man. It was thus a synthesis
of different approaches within the separate disciplines which
compose the wider field of chemotherapy that the Symposium was
concerned.

Those involved in developing new drugs are aware that the
strategy of chemotherapy, all too often, is one of random screening
of potential new compounds, the cost of which has increased alarm-
ingly over recent years. With the knowledge of molecular targets
within the cell and the powerful technique of QSAR analysis screening methods are, however, changing. In this respect a glimpse of
the future was given to us by Dr Tollenaere who demonstrated the
value of knowing the three-dimensional structure of drugs - an
approach which has led to the successful marketing of at least one

drug which was based _ab initio_ upon X-ray crystallographic data analysis of congeners.

A more commonly used approach is that of Hansch or QSAR analysis which, although extremely useful, requires careful choice of the correct physico-chemical and biological parameters. Dr Wardman ably showed that this approach is readily available to all who have access to computing facilities.

Nevertheless, if a new drug is developed and marketed and its mechanism of action known there is every chance that, eventually, resistance will develop - whether to an infecting bacterium or cancer cell and the mechanisms of such resistance in bacteria were reviewed by Professor Smith.

It is only relatively recently that the importance of establishing the mode of action of drugs at the molecular level has been fully realised and this knowledge is paramount in appreciating the selective toxicity of drugs. Even where useful chemotherapeutic agents are not particularly selectively toxic - witness the majority of anticancer drugs as Professor Hellman showed - they may be of potential value elsewhere, as antiprotozoal drugs, or their activity enhanced by an increase in their selectivity of delivery by liposome encapsulation as Dr Gregoriadis illustrated.

Although present anticancer chemotherapy is probably at the level of bacterial chemotherapy at the turn of the century when arsenical drugs were the therapy of choice, new and exciting approaches are bound to make an impact and Dr Stratford convincingly demonstrated the future potential of radiosensitisers in his lecture. However, even when chemotherapy appears to be highly successful, and Dr Willis showed this to be true of anaerobic bacterial infection, there are some areas where effective drugs are noticeably lacking. In antiprotozoal chemotherapy Professor Newton showed that the UNDP/World Bank/WHO special programme for Research and Training in Tropical Diseases has been developed in an attempt to rectify the situation. A similar state of affairs seems to exist in the field of anthelmintic chemotherapy. As Dr Howells pointed out, although novel strategies for helminth control are being actively pursued, the problems of host-parasite relationships are immense and what is needed are new drugs with different targets of action.

In this respect the four major targets of chemotherapeutic action were discussed. Dr Neidle showed that current knowledge of anticancer drugs which bind to DNA can serve as a useful starting point for the rational design of new agents with enhanced activity and/or selective toxicity. Dr Hammond showed that although the membrane can be a selectively toxic target, particularly as regards antifungal agents, the field is hampered by a lack of knowledge of the nature of the target itself. Where DNA is the best characterised target the membrane is the least. The situation, however, is improving as new techniques such as scanning microcalorimetry are being used to probe its structure and function. With the publication in 1965 of the Tipper and Strominger theory of penicillin action, many thought at the time that the mechanism of action of β-lactam antibiotics was solved. It rapidly became apparent that this was not so and Professor Selwyn illustrated the importance of penicillin binding proteins in explaining the action of these drugs - a very active field of continuing research. This is also very true of the ribosome as a target where Dr Cundliffe elegantly showed the way in which antibiotic producer organisms avoid suicide by modifying their own ribosomal RNA.

Whatever field of chemotherapy is considered, be it anticancer, antibacterial or antiprotozoal, and whatever aspect of chemotherapy, be it the drug-target interaction or mechanisms of resistance it is evident that the most useful approach to solving the problems and ultimately create a successful strategy is a multidisciplinary one. This approach does not lack ideas or enthusiasm. Chemotherapy has adopted modern techniques such as the applications of monoclonal antibodies, X-ray crystallography and computer technology faster than any other field of scientific enterprise. It was for these reasons that we hoped that the Symposium would prove valuable in bringing together scientists to compare multidisciplinary approaches in chemotherapy. In this the meeting was a signal success in achieving its objectives.

London, 1982   DIE
                                                                  DRH

3

Antibiotics affecting DNA function

S Neidle

Cancer Research Campaign Biomolecular Structure
Research Group, Department of Biophysics
King's College, 26-29 Drury Lane, London WC2B 5RL

INTRODUCTION

Cancer chemotherapy has as its goals the control, and in favourable cases, even the cure, of the approximately one hundred distinct categories of this disease. The past few years have seen the attainment of these objectives for a small number of cancers, such as acute paediatric leukemia and Hodgkin's disease. Others, including the all-too-common lung and breast cancers, are still relatively unresponsive to drug treatment. Future chemotherapy advances in the clinic will be contingent on new agents having one or more of the factors: increased spectrum of activity, increased cancer versus normal cell selectivity, enhanced anti-tumour activity, and reduced side-effect action. The classic methods of drug development via massive compound screening programmes seem unlikely to achieve these objectives, and thus many laboratories have been engaged in developing more rational approaches.

There are about 20-30 anti-cancer drugs in current clinical use (see for example, Pratt and Ruddon, 1979; Goldin et al., 1981). The majority of these compounds are most active against tumours with rapidly dividing cells. It is thus unsurprising that activity can be attributed to interference with one aspect or other of nucleic acid function, especially of DNA function. Indeed, it is often considered that DNA itself is the most sensitive macromolecular site in a cell. However, this sensitivity necessarily implies that many anti-cancer drugs are relatively non-selective and have general cytotoxic properties. The clinical circumventions of this problem are outside the scope of this paper; suffice it to say that combination chemotherapy using several drugs simultaneously has emerged as a powerful tool in helping to minimise cytotoxic effects.

5

(1)

(2)

(3)

(4)

(5)

(6)

(7)

(8)

Prominent among this small group of clinically-useful drugs are those that are believed to interact directly with the DNA template. In particular, the antibiotics (so-called because of their microbial origin), have attracted wide-spread interest on account of their wide spectrum of activity. Noteworthy examples are daunomycin (4), actinomycin (6), echinomycin (7) and ellipticine (3). In this review, we shall discuss the available evidence describing the interactions of these compounds with DNA, how these relate to activity and indications of some future developments.

DNA as a Drug Receptor

DNA is in many respects one of the best characterised of all biological macromolecules in molecular structural terms. Thus for medicinal chemistry it is an attractive candidate for the study of drug-receptor interactions. The profound progress in DNA sequencing technology is now beginning to advance these studies to a new level of sophistication in proceeding from considerations of DNA-drug interactions as relatively non-specific events, to the establishment of specific loci for these bindings.

The basic features of DNA structure at the atomic level were established by the model-building work of Watson and Crick, and have since been extensively refined by Wilkins and his school. These studies have shown that the basic structure consists of two anti-parallel right-handed helically inter-twined sugar-phosphate strands, which are held together by specific hydrogen-bonding between purine and pyrimidine bases. The complementarity of these 'Watson-Crick' base pairs forms the cornerstone of the genetic code and its expression. Figure 1 shows the structure of the B form of DNA, the polymorph that is believed to predominate under physiological conditions. Other important polymorphs are A-DNA, which resembles double-helical RNA, and the recently-discovered and unexpected left-handed Z-DNA double helix (Wang et al., 1979). B-DNA has ten base pairs per double-helical turn of 360°; thus the rotation per residue is 36°. A-DNA has an eleven-fold helix with a 32.7° rotation per base pair.

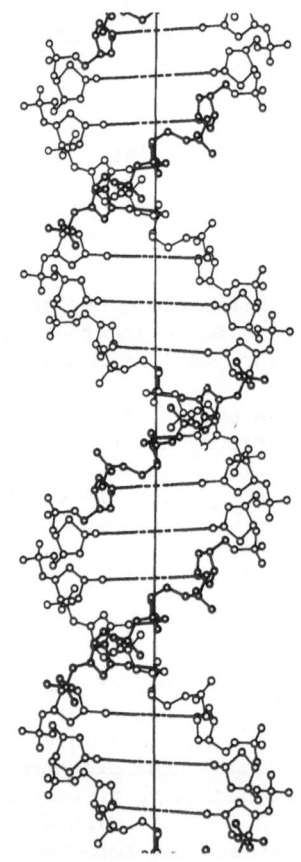

Figure 1. The molecular structure of B-DNA (Courtesy of M.H.F. Wilkins).

For purposes of this discussion, attention will be focussed on the arrangement of the base pairs within the B form. Figure 1 shows that these base pairs are highly planar, and the stacking of adjacent ones at 3.4Å separation is a crucial factor in maintaining the overall stability of the structure. The forces responsible for this stabilisation have been variously termed van der Waals, dispersion or stacking interactions; they are characterised by being relatively non-directional, and having a dependence on the electron polarisation of the molecular species involved. Thus, the heterocyclic bases of DNA are well suited to produce significant stacking stabilisations. The overall arrangement of base pairs in B-DNA may be likened to a stack of coins, linked on the outside by the two sugar-phosphate strands.

Examination of the molecular structures of the antibiotics (3), (4), (6) and (7), as well as of other DNA-binding drugs and mutagens (such as proflavine (1), ethidium (2)), reveals a dominant common feature. This is the possession of a planar heterocyclic aromatic chromophore with dimensions similar to that of a base pair or a pyrimidine base. Recognition of this central feature led directly to the intercalation binding model of Lerman (1961), which has been generally accepted as a major conceptual advance in that it has rationalised and collated a very large body of experimental data.

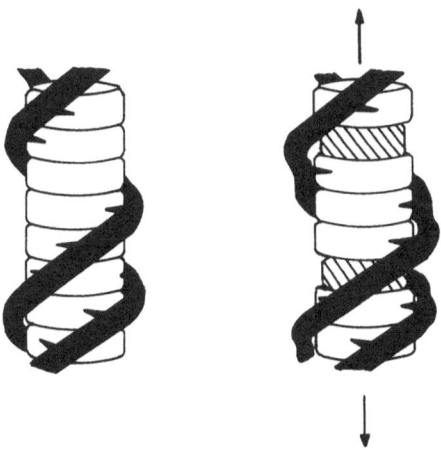

Figure 2. The interaction model, as proposed by Lerman (1961). The left-hand side shows native DNA; on the right hand is seen DNA with bound drug molecules (as shaded discs).

9

The Lerman model (Figure 2) has the planar chromophore of a drug being inserted in between two base pairs, so that for each drug molecule the DNA increases in length by 3.4Å. The model implies an unwinding of the double helix at each site from the 36° value for DNA itself.

The simplicity and all-embracing nature of the model does however imply that a number of aspects of intercalation remain unexplained by it. These have been brought in increasing focus within the past few years, with the realisation that DNA itself is a considerably more complex and subtle molecule than was hitherto suspected. Particularly relevant to this discussion have been the findings that the micro structure of the DNA molecule at any point is dependent on the particular sequence of bases at that point (Dickerson and Drew, 1981). It is now clear that the model of drug interaction presented in Figure 2 cannot address the question of DNA sequence dependence; indeed, the model is unable to define in any way the conformational changes produced in the sugar-phosphate backbone. Most importantly, the model also fails to differentiate between different intercalating drugs, even though effects on DNA, as well as biological ones are often quite distinct.

Biological Effects of Intercalation

The range of biological properties shown by intercalating drugs is wide (reviewed, inter alia, by Gale et al., 1981; Neidle, 1979; Schwartz, 1979; Waring, 1981; Wilson and Jones, 1981), and their consequent clinical and/or laboratory use reflects this diversity. Anti-cancer action has been established for a number of types of intercalator (for example, some acridines and anthracyclines, reviewed in Neidle and Waring (1982)), though by no means all. Anti-bacterial action has been of clinical use, as have anti-parasitic properties. Intercalators produce gross and characteristic changes in cell nuclei appearance. At a sub-cellular level, inhibition of some aspect of nucleic acid synthesis is a sine qua non of intercalation, and is frequently used as a quantitative measure of interaction. Mutagenesis, as detected by a technique such as the Ames test (McCann et al., 1975), is also an invariable property of intercalating compounds.

Both RNA and DNA synthesis are inhibited by compounds such as proflavine (1) and daunomycin (4); for the latter drug, it has been shown in a classic series of experiments (Zunino et al., 1975) that DNA-dependent RNA polymerase inhibition is independent of enzyme concentration, and is thus caused by direct action on the DNA template. Actinomycin D specifically inhibits RNA synthesis. It is not clear whether the intercalated drug for example, blocks the enzyme binding dite, or inhibits strand separation. Kinetic dissociation behaviour of the drug-DNA complex may also be an important factor. Mechanisms of the frame shift type of mutagenesis shown by many intercalators, have frequently been accounted for by the Lerman model, not least because of the historical importance of proflavine-induced frameshifts in establishing the nature of the genetic code (Crick et al., 1961). However, it is now clear that there is as yet no universal model for frameshift mutagenesis which can even qualitatively account for the range of mutating properties shown by intercalating drugs (Neidle, 1979; Drake and Baltz, 1976).

It has recently been established that DNA-intercalating agents characteristically produce single-and double-stranded breaks in DNA, in mammalian cell systems (Ross, Glaubiger and Kohn, 1979; Ross and Bradley, 1981). These breaks are not formed directly by the drugs, but are the result of a consequent susceptibility to enzyme-nicking action. The enzyme(s) responsible may well be topoisomerases (Zwelling et al., 1981), which are activated to an extent that is dependent on the nature of the intercalator. There is, for example, marked difference in strand-break frequency between the two anti-cancer agents m-AMSA (5) and adriamycin (4, with -COMe replaced by -COCH$_2$OH), suggesting that DNA strand breakage is not by itself the cause of the drug's cytotoxic effects.

Physico-chemical Effects of Intercalation

In vitro studies of drug-DNA interaction have been vigorously pursued even prior to the advent of the intercalation model (Lerman, 1961). These have defined and refined many aspects of the model, and play an important role in the evaluation of new drugs, particularly anti-cancer ones. In general, it is now firmly established that the possession of intercalative properties within a series of compounds, is a necessary (though not sufficient in itself) one for anti-cancer activity to be present. Indeed, since activity represents the sum total of many different functions, it would be extremely surprising if intercalative action was a consistently reliable indicator of it, let alone of clinical usefulness. Nonetheless, in vitro evaluations of intercalation into 'naked' DNA can sometimes provide a most significant and useful indicator of anti-neoplastic activity (Table 1).

Binding of drugs to DNA may be conveniently followed by standard spectrophotometric techniques, and binding constants obtained, to a first-order approximation, by Scatchard plot analysis. Typically on binding, the absorption spectrum of the drug in the visible region undergoes a shift to longer wavelengths, (bathochromic shift) and a decrease in absorbance (hypochromic effect). Intercalation association constants are normally in the range $1-5 \times 10^6$ moles^{-1}.

Numerous methods have been used to monitor the changes in DNA structure produced by intercalation (reviewed for example, by

11

Table 1. Biological effects and in vitro binding behaviour of
some daunomycin analogues (Adapted from Neidle, 1978).

	Dose required for 50% inhib- ition of DNA synthesis $(M \times 10^6)$	Average in- crease in survival time as % of controls for ascites tumour	Association constant $(M^{-1} \times 10^6)$	ΔTm in $^\circ C$
Daunomycin	1.6	222	3.8	13.4
Adriamycin	3.4	227	3.0	14.8
N-Acetyl- daunomycin	>8.3	100	1.8×10^2	1.0
4-Demethoxy- daunomycin	1.8	264	2.4	21.0
2-Amino- 2-deoxyglycosyl- daunomycinone	8.8	107	7.1×10^2	8.0
4-Epi- daunomycin	9	234	2.0	12.4

Gale et al., 1981; Neidle, 1978, 1979). Those that demonstrate
an increase in the length of a DNA molecule, for example by
measurement of the viscosity enhancement in sonicated DNA, or
the decrease in sedimentation coefficient on binding a drug, are
especially diagnostic of intercalation.

Probably the most widely-used diagnostic techniques are those
which analyse the unwinding of closed circular super helical DNA;
their development and power owe much to the extensive studies by
Waring and his school (Waring, 1970; Waring, 1981; Gale et al.,
1981). In general, a drug is presumed to bind intercalatively if
it initially removes, and then reverses the handedness of the
supercoiling in such a topologically-constrained DNA. It is possible to determine an unwinding angle per intercalated drug molecule,
which is an estimate of the local unwinding induced by the binding.
These are usually given relative to a value of 26° for ethidium
(Table 2). It is perhaps not always realised that the unwinding
angle parameter at the present time cannot readily be related to
other parameters of intercalation.

The DNA molecule is invariably stabilised upon ligand binding
such that there is an increase in the thermal transition temperature Tm, when DNA undergoes a helix → coil transition. The resulting Δ Tm value has often (though erroneously) been taken as proof
of intercalation. Nonetheless, this easily-measured quantity has

Table 2.   Unwinding angles for various intercalating drugs (from
          Waring, 1981).

Proflavine	(1)	17°	Actinomycin D	(6)	26°
Ethidium	(2)	26°	Echinomycin	(7)	48°
Ellipticine	(3)	17°	Diacridine with		
Daunomycin	(4)	11°	$R-(CH_2)_6$	(8)	33°
M-AMSA	(5)	21°			

frequently been used as a rough guide to the relative strength of
intercalative binding for series of anti-cancer drug analogues.
Comparisions between Δ Tm studies in different laboratories should
be made with care as both Δ Tm and Tm values are markedly ionic-
strength-dependent (as indeed is the intercalation process itself).

Nuclear magnetic resonance spectroscopy is emerging as a powerful technique for studying drug-DNA interactions in solution,
which can provide kinetic and thermodynamic parameters. In addition, NMR is capable of in principle yielding the most detailed
structural and conformational data, although in practise it has not
as yet been possible to fully defined the geometry of an intercalative interaction at this level using the method. It has been
shown that the ring-current chemical shifts induced in the protons
bonded to a drug chromophore, upon intercalation between adjacent
base pairs, are characteristic of this process, and may thus be
taken as a quantitative indication of intercalation (Patel, 1979).

Specificity of Binding

All of these methods of probing the drug-DNA intercalative
processes are, with the exception of NMR, relatively coarse-grained
ones in that they do not provide information on the differences in
the binding at different sequences, but instead tend to average
these out. Thus for example, to discuss different drugs solely in
terms of binding constants for calf thymus DNA, may be very mis-
leading. There are several firm lines of evidence that intercalation is a sequence-dependent process, whose nature is dependent
on the steric and electronic properties of the drug vis a vis its
preferred sequence of base pairs. Thus, even simple intercalators
such as ethidium and proflavine display a marked preference for
pyrimidine-3',5'-purine sequences (Reinhardt and Krugh, 1978; Patel
and Canuel, 1977). Actinomycin D (6) has a very selective requirement for a 2-amino purine residue (such as guanine) at the 5' side
of its intercalation site, which is due to a specific pattern of
hydrogen bonding between this base and the threonine residues of
the drug's pentapeptides (Takusagawa et al., 1982). In general,
increased specificity is paralleled by increases in the complexity
of the molecular structure of an intercalating drug. Thus, echinomycin (7), like actinomycin D, selectively inhibits DNA-dependent

RNA polymerase. Echinomycin binds 2-3 times more strongly to the synthetic poly nucleotide poly (dG-dC) than to poly (dA-dT), whereas its analogue triosin A, (differing by having an extra sulphur atom in the central peptide cross bridge), shows a reversal of this order (Wakelin and Waring, 1976; Gale et al., 1981). The synthetic analogue 'tandem', des-N-tetramethyl triosin A, binds co-operatively to poly (dA-dT) and barely at all to poly (dG-dC); plausible explanations at the molecular level have been advanced for this extreme behaviour (Viswamitra et al., 1981).

Echinomycin and its analogues are examples of bis-intercalating agents, which interact simultaneously at two binding sites. Since in general intercalation at any one site excludes neighbouring sites from binding a drug molecule, bifunctional binding must follow the model shown in Figure 3(a), and not that in (b). Echinomycin accordingly has its planar chromophores spaced 10.2 Å apart. Selectivity in DNA interaction with such compounds has been demonstrated with a bis analogue of ethidium which inhibits restriction enzyme cutting of a plasmid in a sequence-dependent manner (Ibeda and Dervan, 1982).

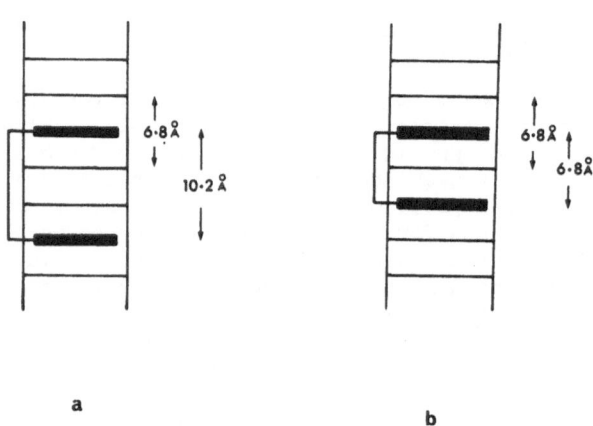

a   b

Figure 3.   Schematic illustration of bifunctional intercalation into DNA.   In (a), neighbour exclusion binding is shown in contrast to the violation situation in (b).

Structure - activity Relationships

There have been very many studies on the systematic examination of DNA-intercalation properties in relation to activity parameters, for many series of drug analogues. Anthracyclines,
ellipticines, acridines and actinomycins have perhaps been most
extensively investigated; in this section we shall highlight just
a few such reports. The anti-cancer activity and DNA-binding
ability of the anthracycline drugs (typified by daunomycin), are
markedly dependent upon retention of stereochemistry for the amino-
sugar moiety (Table 1) (Di Marco and Arcamone, 1975; Henry, 1975;
Brown, 1978; Neidle, 1978). Removal of the methoxy group on the
aromatic ring would be expected to increase intercalative ability;
this has indeed been found (Zunino, Di Marco and Zaccara, 1979),
and is accompanied by a corresponding improvement in experimental
anti-tumour activity. This compound has certain clinical advantages compared to the parent drug, and is currently in clinical
trial.

Daunomycin and adriamycin, in spite of their undoubted high
efficacy, have a number of associated problems. They produce
severe cumulative dose-related cardiotoxicity; they are expensive
drugs, and they are difficult to modify chemically. For these
reasons, there have been a number of attempts at establishing
simple DNA-binding analogues, all of which have used anthraquinones
(Figure 4) as starting-points.

The compound with $R^1 = R^2 = -NHCH_2CH_2NHCH_2CH_2OH$ and $R^3 = R^4 =$
OH (Murdock et al., 1979; Johnson et al., 1979) has received particular attention in that it seems as least as active as adriamycin

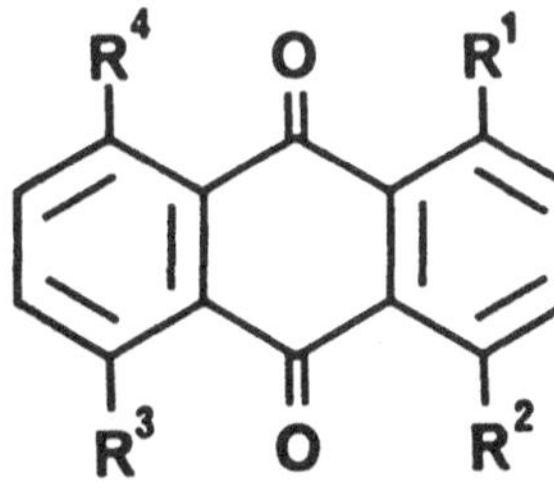

Figure 4. The anthraquinone ring system, with positions of substitution shown that are of current interest for anti-cancer compounds.

against several experimental tumour systems; preliminary clinical
trial data has recently been obtained, and is most promising.
The series in general shows a strong causal relationship between
interaction with DNA and activity. However, since most of the
reported studies rely on Δ Tm measurements for estimating the
former, it is unsurprising that the relationships are sometimes
less than perfect.

Acridines have probably had more attention as intercalating
and mutagenic agents than any other class of compound, and indeed
the knowledge that acridine orange and its cogeners bind to cell
nuclei predates the Watson-Crick model for DNA by many years. It
is however, only recently, that their potential anti-tumour
activity has received systematic attention, largely as a result of
the work of Cain and his colleagues. Their monumental studies on
many hundreds of 9-anilinoacridines have established that m-AMSA
(5) has high activity and much promise. It has, for example, been
demonstrated that there is a quantitative relationship between DNA-
binding constants and dose potency in L1210 tests (Baguley et al.,
1981a), and between binding and molecular structure (Baguely et
al., 1981b). QSAR relationships have also been extensively used
in this series to establish further cross-correlations with other
important variables such as hydrophobicity (Denny et al., 1982).

STRUCTURAL ASPECTS OF INTERCALATION

X-ray crystallography has been extensively employed to define
the details of intercalation geometry at the atomic level, thereby
providing information at a defined site. To date, the molecular
structures of some dozen drug-dinucleoside complexes have been reported (summarised by Neidle, 1981a,b; Neidle and Berman, 1982).
The range of drugs in these is considerable; proflavine has been
especially studied (Neidle et al., 1977, 1978; Shieh et al., 1980;
Neidle, Berman and Shieh, 1980) as well as for example actinomycin
D, ellipticine, ethidium and acridine orange (Jain, Tsai and Sobell,
1977; Takusagawa et al., 1982). These model systems have duplex
Watson-Crick base-paired structures with intercalated drug only
when the sequence of the dinucleoside is pyrimidine-3',5'-purine;
in other cases, such as with ApA and proflavine (Neidle et al.,
1978) or d(GpC) and actinomycin D (Takusagawa et al., 1982), the
dinucleoside adopts an extended, opened-out conformation. Thus,
these systems provide further evidence for sequence-preference
binding.

The complexes with double-helical-like features are typified
by that shown in Figure 5. The backbone is extended so as to make
top and bottom base pairs 6.8Å apart. It is perhaps surprising
that the detailed conformation of the backbone is very similar in
all these complexes, and therefore does not depend on the nature

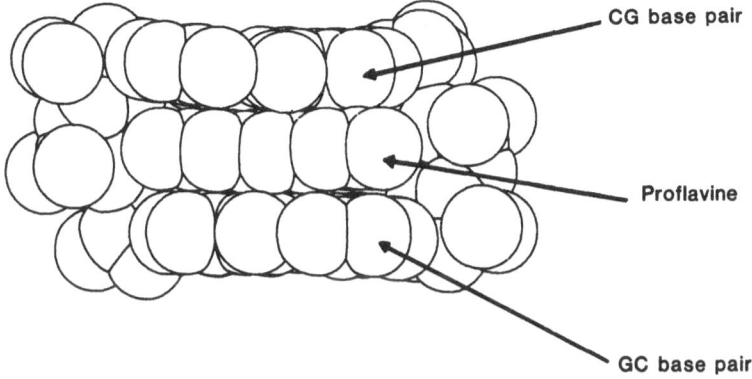

CG base pair

Proflavine

GC base pair

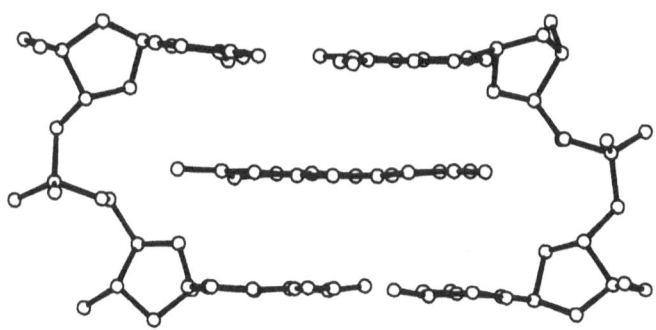

Figure 5. The molecular structure of the d(CpG)-proflavine complex, shown in both van der Waals and ball-and-stick represen-
tations. (Data from Shieh et al., 1980).

of the intercalated drug (Berman, Neidle and Stodola, 1978).
Furthermore, this invariant property produces structures which
are closely related to A-rather than B-form nucleic acids. It
appears that the nature and size of the drug itself is manifest

in differences in base-pair hydrogen-bonding geometry, and in base-pair twist and tilt (Shieh et al., 1980). These distinctions between the structures are the primary cause of the observed differences in apparent unwinding angle, a topic which in the past has excited some controversy. Thus, the ethidium-5-iodo-CpG complex (Jain, Tsai and Sobell, 1977) has an unwinding angle of 26°, in seeming agreement with the measurements on this drug bound to closed circular DNA. By contrast, the proflavine-CpG complex has a 0° unwinding angle (Neidle et al., 1977). In truth, these angles, which should be more correctly termed base-turn angles, merely reflect characteristics of the model systems, and should not be taken as representative of intercalation into polymeric DNAs. It is much more likely that unwinding is actually distributed over several residues, as has been found in a daunomycin-hexanucleotide complex (Quigley et al., 1980). This structure also displays 0° 'unwinding' at the actual site of binding.

The extent to which these drug-dinucleoside intercalation structures actually model all the details of intercalation into DNA itself remains undetermined, although it is clear that many of the important aspects are indeed paralleled in the two types of system. The structural questions remaining to be answered, especially concerning conformational changes in adjacent residues and their sequence dependence, must await X-ray crystallographic studies on complexes with larger length oligonucleotide. Even so, it is possible at the present time to conceive of utilising the information now available, for purposes of drug design.

Model-building Studies

The unique backbone geometry for drug intercalation into a dinucleoside can be derived directly from A-form nucleic acids by means of torsion angle changes at the O5'-C5' bond and 3'-end glycosidic angle. Figure 6 shows a resultant atomic arrangement, with the drug binding site readily apparent. Procedures for systematically fitting a molecule into a receptor site are actively being developed in a number of laboratories. The approach adopted in this context by several groups, including our own, involves the simultaneous use of interactive computer graphics and empirical energy calculations (Dearing, Weiner and Kollman, 1981; Islam et al., 1982; Miller and Newlin, 1982). The procedures involve the location of a minimum-energy position for a particular drug molecule; modifications to the structure, for example by varying substitution patterns can then be systematically studied for their effects on the energy of the interaction and its geometry. In this way, it may well be possible to systematically design an optimally-binding drug analogue suitable for further in vitro and in vivo study. Among the advantages of this approach for the study of drug-receptor interactions, are that (i) detailed structural and energetic information can be readily obtained (ii) the site studied can be one of

18

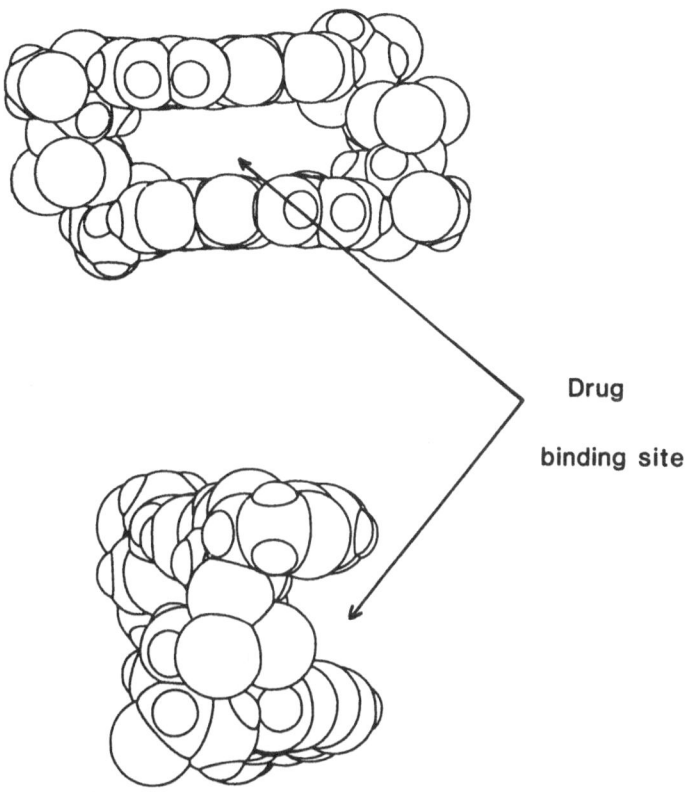

Drug

binding site

Figure 6. Two views of the generalised intercalator receptor geometry, for the CG sequence.

preferred binding and (iii) it is straight forward and speedy to investigate large numbers of drug analogues.

EPILOGUE

The intercalation concept, after twenty-one years of continuing existence, is now moving away from its original relatively-undefined and non-specific role. By increasingly focussing on sequence-specificy and preference, and examining these sites in more detail, the subject is entering a new era of understanding and indeed usefulness. Information at these more detailed levels will be of relevance not only to rational drug design, but also to studies on the nature of site-specific mutagenesis and repair.

References

Baguley, B.C., Denny, W.A., Atwell, G.J. and Cain, B.F. (1981a). Potential Antitumour Agents. 25. Quantitative Relationships between Antitumour (L1210) Potency and DNA Binding for 4'-(9-Acridinylamino)methanesulfon-m-aniside Analogues. J. Med. Chem., 24, 520-525.

Baguley, B.C., Denny, W.A., Atwell, G.J. and Cain, B.F. (1981b). Potential Antitumour Agents. 34. Quantitative Relationships between DNA Binding and Molecular Structure for 9-Anilinoacridines Substituted in the Anilino Ring. J. Med. Chem., 24, 170-177-

Berman, H.M., Neidle, S. and Stodola, R.K. (1978). Drug-nucleic Acid Interactions: Confromational Flexibility at the Intercalation Site. Proc. natl. Acad. Sci. USA, 75, 828-832.

Brown, J.R. (1978). Adriamycin and Related Anthracycline Antibiotics. Prog. Med. Chem., 15m 125-164.

Crick, F.H.C., Barnett, L., Brenner, S. and Watts-Tobin, R.J. (1961). General Nature of the Genetic Code for Proteins. Nature, Lond., 192, 1227-1232.

Dearing, A., Weiner, P. and Kollman, P.A. (1981). Molecular Mechanical Studies of Proflavine and Acridine Orange Intercalation. Nucleic Acids Res., 9, 1483-1497.

Denny, W.A., Cain, B.F., Atwell, G.J., Hansch, C., Panthananickal, A. and Leo, A. (1982). Potential Antitumour Agents. 36. Quantitative Relationships between Experimental Antitumour Activity and Structure for the General Class of 9-Anilinoacridine Antitumour Agents. J. Med. Chem., 25, 276-315.

Dickerson, R.E. and Drew, H.R. (1981). Structure of a B-DNA Dodecamer II Influence of Base Sequence on Helix Structure. J. molec. Biol., 149, 761-786.

Di Marco, A. and Arcamone, F. (1975). DNA Complexing Antibiotics: Daunomycin, Adriamycin and their Derivatives. Arzneim.-Forsch. 25, 368-375.

Drake, J.W. and Baltz, R.H. (1974). The Biochemistry of Mutagenesis. Ann. Rev. Biochem., 45, 11-37.

Gale, E.F., Cundliffe, E., Reynolds, P.E., Richmond, M.H. and Waring, M.J. (1981). The Molecular Basis of Antibiotic Action, 2nd Ed. John Wiley, London.

Goldin, A., Venditti, J.M., MacDonald, J.S., Muggiam F.M., Henney, J.E. and DeVita, V.T. (1981). Current Results of the Screening

Program at the Division of Cancer Treatment, National Cancer Institute. Eur. J. Cancer, 17, 129-142.

Henry, D.W. (1976). Adriamycin, in Cancer Chemotherapy (ed. A. Sartorelli) American Chemical Society, Washington.

Ikeda, R.A. and Dervan, P.B. (1982). Sequence-Selective Inhibition of Restriction Endonucleases by the Polyintercalator Bis(methidium) Spermine. J. amer. Chem. Soc. 104, 296-197.

Islam, S.A., Kuroda, R., Neidle, S., Brown, J.R., Gandecha, B.M. and Patterson, L.H. (1982). Computer Graphics in Rational Anti-Cancer Drug Design. Biochem. Soc. Trans., in press.

Jain, S.C., Tsai, C.C. and Sobell, H.M. (1977). Visualisation of Drug.-Nucleic Acid Interactions at Atomic Resolution II Structure of Ethidium/Dinucleoside Monophosphate Crystalline Complex, Ethidium: 5-Iodocytidylyl (3'-5') Guanosine. J. molec. Biol., 114, 317-331.

Johnson, R.K., Zee-Cheng, R.K.Y., Lee, W.W., Acton, E.M., Henry, D.W. and Cheng, C.C. (1979). Experimental Antitumour Activity of Aminoanthraquinones. Cancer Treatment Reports, 63m 425-439.

Lerman, L.S. (1961). Structural Considerations in the Interactions of DNA and Acridines. J. molec. Biol., 3, 18-30.

McCann, J., Choi, E., Yamasaki, E. Ames, B.N. (1975). Definition of Carcinogens as Mutagens in the Salmonella/microsome Test: Assay of 300 chemicals. Proc. natl. Acad. Sci. USA, 72, 5135-5139.

Miller, K.J. & Newlin, D.D. (1982) Interactions of Molecules with Nucleic Acids. Vl. Computer Design of Chromophoric Intercalating Agents. Biopolymers, 21, 633-652.

Murdock, K.C., Child, R.G., Fabio, P.F., Angier, R.B., Wallace, R.E., Durr, F.E. and Citarella, R.V. (1979). Antitumour Agents. 1. 1,4-Bis[(aminoalkyl)amino]-9,10-anthracenediones. J. Med. Chem., 22, 1024-1030.

Neidle, S. (1978). Interactions of Daunomycin and Related Anti-biotics with Biological Receptors, in Topics in Antibiotic Chem-istry, Vol. 2 (ed. P.G. Sammes). Ellis Horwood, Chichester, pp. 239-278.

Neidle, S. (1979). The Molecular Basis for the Action of Some DNA-Binding Drugs. Prog. Med. Chem., 16m 151-221.

Neidle, S. (1981a). Structural Studies on the Interactions of Nucleic Acids with Drugs and Mutagens. Comments. Mol. Cell Biophys. 1, 171-188.

Neidle, S. (1981b). Oligonucleotide and Polynucleotide-Drug Complexes in the Crystalline State, in <u>Topics in Nucleic Acid Structure</u>. (ed. S. Neidle) MacMillan Press, London.

Neidle, S. Achari, A., Taylor, G.L., Berman, H.M., Carrell, H.L., Glusker, J.P. and Stallings, W. C. (1977). Structure of a Dinucleoside Phosphate-Drug Complex as Model for Nucleic Acid-Drug Interaction. Nature, Lond., <u>269</u>, 304-307.

Neidle, S. and Berman, H.M. (1982). Drug Intercalation in Nucleic Acids: The Current State of Knowledge. <u>In Molecular Structure and Biological Activity</u>. (eds. J.F. Griffin and W.L. Duax), Elsevier, New York, in the press.

Neidle, S., Berman, H.M. and Shieh, H.S. (1980). Highly Structured Water Network in Crystals of a Deoxydinucleoside-drug Complex. Nature, Lond., <u>288</u>, 129-133.

Neidle, S., Taylor, G., Sanderson, M., Shieh, H.S. and Berman, H.M. (1978). A 1:2 Crystalline Complex of ApA: Proflavine: a Model for Binding to Single-stranded Regions in RNA. Nucleic Acids Res. <u>5</u>, 4417-4422.

Neidle, S. and Waring, M.J. (eds.) (1982). <u>Molecular Aspects of Anti-Cancer Drug Action</u>. MacMillan Press, London, in the press.

Patel, D.J. (1979). Nuclear Magnetic Resonance Studies of Drug-Nucleic Acid Interactions at the Synthetic DNA level in Solution. Acc. Chem. Res., <u>12</u>, 118-125

Patel, D.J. and Canuel, L.L. (1977). Sequence Specificity of Mutagen-Nucelic Acid Complexes in Solution:Intercalation and Mutagen-Base Pair Overlap Geometries for Proflavine Binding to dC-dC-dG-dG and dG-dG-dC-dC Self-complementary Duplexes. Proc. natl.Acad. Sci. USA, <u>74</u>, 2624-2628.

Pratt, W.B. and Ruddon, R.W. (1979) <u>The Anticancer Drugs</u>. Oxford University Press, New York.

Quigley, G.J., Wang, A.H.-J., Ughetto, G., van der Marel, G., van Boom, J.H. and Rich, A. (1980). Molecular Structure of an Anti-cancer Drug-DNA Complex:Daunomycin plus (dCpGpTpApCpG). Proc. natl. Acad. Sci. USA <u>77</u>, 7204-7208.

Reinhardt, C.G. and Krugh, T.R. (1978). A Comparative Study of Ethidium Bromide Complexes with Dinucleotides and DNA:Direct Evidence for Intercalation and Nucleic Acid Sequence Preferences. Biochemistry, <u>17</u>, 4845-4854.

Schwartz, H.S. (1979). Biochemical Action and Selectivity of Intercalating Drugs. Adv. Cancer Chemotherapy, <u>1</u>, 1-60.

Shieh, H.S., Berman, H.M., Dabrow, M. and Neidle, S. (1980). The Structure of a Drug-deoxydinucleoside phosphate Complex:Generalised Conformational Behaviour of Intercalation Complexes with RNA and DNA Fragments. Nucleic Acids Res., 8 85-97.

Takusagawa, F., Dabrow, M., Neidle, S. and Berman, H.M. (1982). The Structure of a Pseudo Intercalated Complex between Actinomycin and the DNA Binding Sequence d(GpC). Nature, Lond., 296, 466-469.

Viswamitra, M.A., Kennard, O., Cruse, W.B.T., Egert, E., Sheldrick, G.M., Jones, P.G., Waring, M.J., Wakelin, L.P.G. and Olsen, R.K. (1981). Structure of Tandem and its Implication for Bifunctional Intercalation into DNA. Nature, Lond., 289, 817-819.

Wakelin, L.P.G. and Waring, M.J. (1976). The Binding of Echinomycin to Deoxyribonucleic Acid. Biochem. J., 157, 721-740.

Wang, A.H.-J., Quigley, G.J., Kolpak, F.J., Crawford, J.L., van Boom, J.H., van der Marel, G. and Rich, A. (1979). Molecular Structure of a Left-handed Double-helical DNA Fragment at Atomic Resolution. Nature Lond., 282, 680-686.

Waring, M.J. (1970). Variation of the Supercoils in Closed Circular DNA by Binding of Antibiotics and Drugs:Evidence for Molecular Models Involving Intercalation. J. molec. Biol., 54, 247-279.

Waring, M.J. (1981). DNA Modification and Cancer. Ann. Rev. Biochem., 50, 159-192.

Wilson, W.D. and Jones, R.L. (1981). Intercalating Drugs:DNA Binding and Molecular Pharmacology. Adv. Pharmac. Chemotherapy, 18, 177-222.

Zunino, F., Di Marco, A. and Zaccara A. (1979). Molecular Structural Effects Involved in the Interaction of Anthracyclines with DNA. Chem.-Biol. Interactions, 24, 217-225.

Zunino, F., Gambetta, R., Di Marco, A., Zaccara, A. and Luoni, G. (1975). A comparison of the Effects of Daunomycin and Adriamycin on Various DNA Polymerases. Cancer Res., 35, 754-760.

Zwelling, L.A., Michaels, S., Erickson, L.C., Ungerleider, R.S., Nichols, M. and Kohn, K.W. (1981). Protein-associated Deoxyribonucleic Acid Strand Breaks in L1210 Cells Treated with the Deoxyribonucleic Acid Intercalating Agents 4'-(9-Acridinylamino) methanesulfon-m-anisidide and Adriamycin. Biochemistry, 20, 6553-6563.

Antimicrobial agents affecting
membrane function

S M Hammond

Department of Microbiology, University of Leeds
Leeds, LS2 9JT, UK

Although biological membranes are generally impermeable they contain components which can permit or catalyse the translocation of specific solutes between the two sides of the membrane. Hence the membrane represents a region of chemical anisotrophy between two phases of different chemical composition. This means that the membrane experiences mechanical stress through differences in pressure across the membrane's thickness and this sets up corresponding tensions in the plane of the membrane. The unique physical and biological properties exhibited by biological membranes make the components that constitute bacterial membranes very distinct from other cellular materials. Pure cytoplasmic membrane constitutes approximately 10% of total cell weight, mainly protein (50-70%) and lipid (20-30%) depending on species (Rogers, et al 1980).

The main class of lipid present in bacterial membranes is phospholipid. Gram-positive bacteria contain many types of phospholipid; phosphatidylglycerol, phosphatidylethanolamine, diphosphatidylglycerol and aminoacylphosphatidylglycerol while the membranes of Gram-negative bacteria consist mainly of phosphatidylethanolamine. Fungal membranes differ from those of prokaryotes in that they contain appreciable amounts of sterol, mainly ergosterol. Some of the membrane proteins are easily removed by simple aqueous washing and these are believed to be surface epiproteins with an essentially hydrophilic character. Others can be only extracted using organic solvents and are thought to be buried deep in the hydrophobic membrane core. The cytoplasmic membrane contains the enzymes of the cytochrome chain and energy transduction, enzymes responsible for metabolite transport and is the site of synthesis of cell wall, extramural and membrane components and of extracellular protein toxins.

Complex biochemical processes such as energy transduction and
envelope biosynthesis require co-ordinated participation of
diverse molecular species and may only occur efficiently if all
the components are held in close proximity.   The intimate
relationship existing between the lipid and protein components of
the cell membrane provide this necessary micro-environment.

Many antimicrobial agents have been shown to disturb the
function of the microbial cytoplasmic membrane and because of the
vital role the membrane plays in the organisms physiology, such
compounds exhibit high potency and rapid antimicrobial action
(Lambert 1978).   However few of the many membrane active antimicrobials described have become effective chemotherapeutic
agents.   The minimal selective toxicity properties shown by the
majority of membrane active drugs is believed to be an inevitable
consequence of the intrinsic similarity between prokaryote and
eukaryote membranes.   In the main, membrane active antimicrobials
are used as antiseptics and their use within the body restricted
to a small number of applications where, although not ideal on
toxicological grounds, they remain the only effective therapy.
However with increased understanding of the structure and function
of membranes and rational drug design, the development of novel
membrane active drugs is now undergoing something of a renaissance.

It is convenient to divide drugs acting upon the microbial
membrane into three groups; agents which perturb the membrane's
selective permeability properties, inhibitors of energy
transduction and drugs which interfere with the biosynthetic
capacity of the membrane.   Since all the metabolic functions of
the cytoplasmic membrane are closely related, effects consequent
upon the primary action of the drug may often be observed, for
example ionophore antibiotics markedly increase the cation
permeability of the membrane, which under certain conditions can
uncouple oxidative phosphorylation in the organism preventing
the generation of energy.   Similarly, the effect of the agent may
change with drug concentration.

AGENTS WHICH DESTROY THE SELECTIVE PERMEABILITY
PROPERTIES OF THE MEMBRANE.

Agents which damage the membranes permeability barrier may be
detected by monitoring the release of low molecular weight
components into the medium following drug exposure.   The loss of
purine and pyrimidine-containing compounds can be determined by
monitoring the release of 260nm absorbing material; amino acids,

sugars, cations and phosphate by chemical electrochemical or radio-isotope methods (Russell, Morris and Allwood 1973, Hammond and Lambert 1973).

Phenols

Halogenated derivatives of phenols, cresols and xylenol elicit the release of low molecular weight material from bacteria. Such compounds, including "Lysol" and "Dettol", appear to denature membrane proteins and at high concentrations induce lysis.

Detergents

Two catonic detergents cetyltrimethyl ammonium bromide (CTAB) and cetylpyridium chloride (CPC) are potent bacteriocides and being well tolerated by mammalian tissues have found extensive use as skin-sterilizing agents and in antiseptic lozenges.

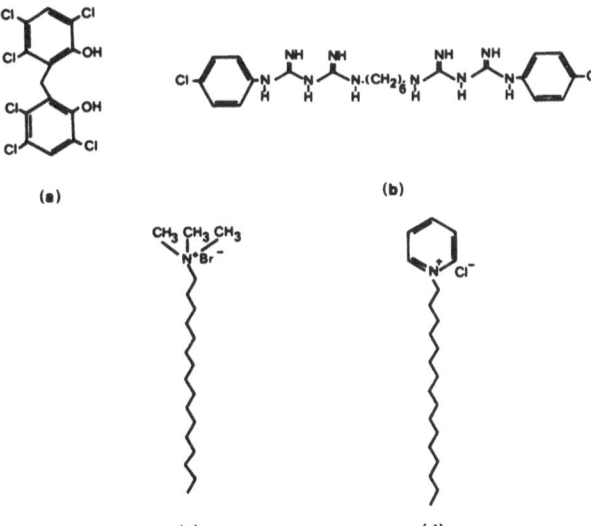

Fig. 1. Structure of membrane-active antiseptics: phenol antiseptics (a) hexachlorophene; cationic antiseptics (b) chlorhexidine, (c) cetyltrimethyl ammonium bromide, (d) cetylpyridium chloride.

27

Anionic detergents are less effective bacteriocides than their cationic equivalents. Non-ionic detergents have little anti-microbial action. The positively charged head groups of the cationic detergents bind to the phosphate head groups of the membrane phospholipid and the alkyl chains penetrate the hydrophobic interior of the membrane (Hugo 1971, Helenius and Simmons 1975). The antibacterial activity of alkyl quaternary ammonium bromides increases with the lengthening of the alkyl chain from C_6 to C_{16} (Fig. 2). With the increase in alkyl chain length the water solubility of the compound falls, lipid solubility rises and surface active properties become more marked. The ability of the agent to penetrate the hydrophobic core of the membrane and to destroy the permeability barrier appear to depend upon the length of the side chain (Figure 2). Smith et al (1975).

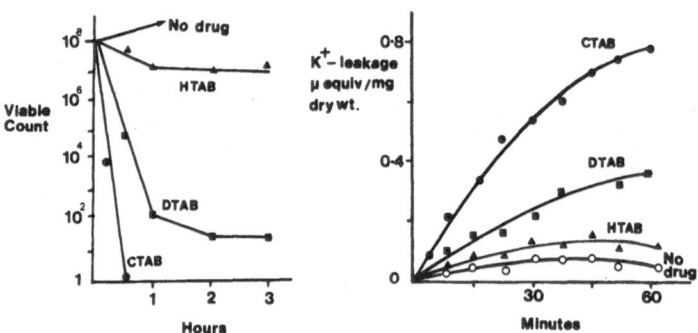

Fig. 2. Effect of alkyl chain length upon the antimicrobial properties of alkyl quaternary ammonium bromides. Escherichia coli was exposed to equimolar (50μm) concentrations of hexyltrimethyl ammonium bromide (HTAB) $C_6H_{13}N^+(CH_3)_3Br^-$, dodecyltrimethyl ammonium bromide (DTAB) $C_{12}H_{25}N^+(CH_3)_3Br^-$ and cetyltrimethyl ammonium bromide (CTAB $C_{16}H_{33}N^+(CH_3)Br^-$ and the number of survivors determined. The release of intracellular potassium by 50μM CTAB, DTAB or HTAB was monitored using a K^+-selective electrode.

Chlorhexidine, 1, 6-di(4 chlorophenyl diguanidino) hexane is used widely in medicine and veterinary practice as a topical agent. The mechanism of action of the drug depends upon the concentration applied. The cationic nature of the agent permits it to bind to negative groups on the cell surface. Low concentrations (5µg ml^{-1}) inhibit the membrane bound ATPase of <u>Streptococcus faecalis</u>, thereby halting energy-dependent processes such as cation transport (Harold <u>et al</u> 1969). Slightly higher concentrations (10-100µg ml^{-1}) produce rapid leakage of cytoplasmic components but at concentrations above 100µg ml^{-1} the rate of cytoplasmic leakage diminishes, presumably due to the reaction of chlorhexidine with cytoplasmic components, mainly protein and nucleic acids, to form a precipitate, which effectively seals the cell.

Cyclic Polypeptide Antibiotics

The cyclic polypeptide antibiotics can be divided into two groups on the basis of the number of amino acids constituting the peptide ring. The cyclic decapeptides, including the tyrocidins and gramicidin S, contain a number of non-polar amino acids and one or two free amino groups. The left hand portion of the decapeptide ring is common to all members of the group, the right hand portion is variable (Fig. 3). Tyrocidin, produced by <u>Bacillus brevis</u>, is more active against Gram-positive than Gram-negative bacteria, the lethal action being the direct result of a generalised disruption of the cell membrane and leakage of cellular material. The surface active properties of cyclic polypeptide antibiotics and the ability to form micelles in aqueous solution appear to be crucial to the bactericidal properties of the drug. Linear analogues of identical amino acid sequence fail to exhibit activity. The presence of non-polar amino acids (Pro, Leu, Val and Phe) and basic amino acids (Asp, Orn and Phe) seem essential for activity. The hydrophobic non-polar residues appear to anchor the molecule to the membrane and the basic amino groups disturb the ionic interactions between membrane components.

The second group, the polymyxins, consist of a series of chemically related cyclic antibiotics produced by <u>Bacillus</u> species. They are composed of a cyclic heptapeptide moiety containing four molecules of diaminobutyric acid, one of which bears a peptide side chain, terminating in a fatty acid residue (Fig. 3). This structure has been compared to that of the cationic detergents, with the cyclic heptapeptide bearing free amino groups providing the positively-charged hydrophilic head and the side chain, containing the fatty acid substituent, providing a hydrophobic tail. Aqueous solutions of polymyxin are strongly surface-active and the effects upon bacteria are identical to those elicited by cationic

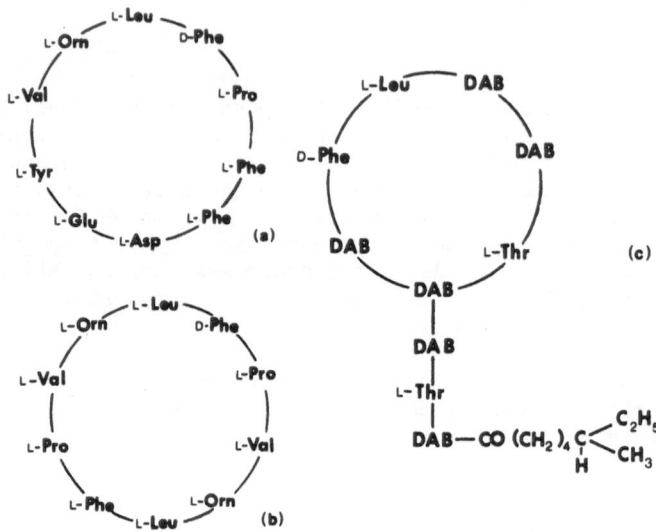

Fig. 3. Cyclic polypeptide antibiotics (a) tyrocidin A,
(b) gramicidin S and polymyxin B . Constituent amino
acids are leucine (Leu), phenylalanine (Phe), proline (Pro),
asparagine (Asp), glutamine (Glu), tyrosine (Tyr), valine
(Val), ornithine (Orn) and 2,4-diaminobutyric acid (DAB).

detergents, i.e loss of cellular components and precipitation of
the cytoplasm.   The amino groups of 2, 4 diaminobutyric acid and
the side chain are both essential for antibacterial action, since
their removal reduces activity.   It is believed that free amino
groups on the cyclic polypeptide portion of the molecule associate
with the phosphate and amino groups of phosphatidylethanolamine
head groups in the membrane and participate in a reaction involving
a mutual transfer of protons between the charged groups.   This
creates a change in the charge distribution in the membrane and a
general breakdown of membrane organisation.

Polymyxins are chiefly active against Gram-negative bacteria,
particularly against Pseudomonad infections.   Although the drugs
exhibit nephrotoxicity, polymyxins are the only membrane active
drugs which possess sufficient selective toxicity towards bacterial
membranes to be of clinical use.

Ionophore and Channel-forming Antibiotics

Ionophores are a group of both cyclic and linear polypeptide
antibiotics which share the ability to facilitate the passage of
inorganic ions across biological membrane.   Although because of
their high toxicity towards both mammalian cells and bacteria,

ionophores are of little use in treating microbial infections in man, these compounds have proved valuable tools in the study of membrane transport processes.

Valinomycin, the ionophore which has received the most attention, is a cyclic depsipeptide, in which the members of the ring are arranged in alternating pairs of D and L configurations. Enniatin B is a smaller cyclic peptide with a 9-membered ring. Valinomycin and enniatin B contain no charged groups and are classed as neutral ionophores. Carboxylic ionophores, such as monensin and nigericin, are linear antibiotics containing oxygenated heterocyclic residues with a single carboxyl group at the end of the chain.

Ionophores have the unique ability to form lipid-soluble complexes with metal ions. Valinomycin shows a high affinity for potassium ions; this ability depending entirely on the alternation of D and L pairs, and change in conformation destroying complex formation (Fig. 4). Other cations, e.g. sodium can also complex with valinomycin, but their smaller size makes the complex less stable. It is thought that the lipophilic ionophore-cation complex shuttles across the membrane, moving ions from regions of high, to regions of low ion concentration.

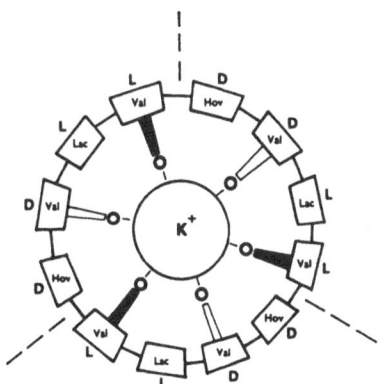

Fig. 4. Structure of the valinomycin-potassium complex. In the valinomycin ring the three residues are valine (Val), 2-hydroxy-isovaleric acid (Hov) and lactic acid (Lac). The dotted lines separate the repeating units and the asymmetric centres are labelled D or L. The central cation (K^+) is co-ordinated by 6 oxygen atoms derived from carbonyl groups of valine residues.

The gramicidins and alamethicin have been termed "quasi-ionophores" since they facilitate the passage of ions across the membrane, not by carrying them in the form of lipid-soluble complexes, but by creating channels in the membrane.
Gramicidins A, B and C (but not S) are linear peptide antibiotics exhibiting very similar antimicrobial properties to valinomycin. Gramicidin A dissolves in the membrane, dimerised in a head to head association forming a spiral structure spanning the membrane with a central hydrophilic pore capable of acting as an ion conducting channel.

Alamethicin is a cyclic peptide antibiotic, containing 18 amino acid residues, which form lipid soluble cation complexes. The conductance it induces in membranes varies with applied potential and it has been suggested that a stack of 6 drug molecules combine to form the conducting channel (Lambert 1978).

Polyene Antifungal Antibiotics

The polyene antibiotic group consists of a series of macrocyclic ring compounds produced by Streptomyces sp., which although potent antifungal agents show no antibacterial activity. The macrolide ring of the polyene antibiotic consists of two very distinct parts (Fig. 5); the first is a series of conjugated double bonds, which gives the group its name.

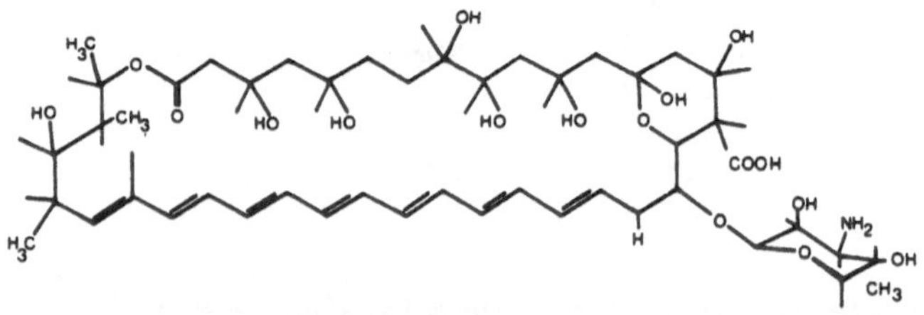

Fig. 5.   Structure of amphotericin B.

32

Polyene antibiotics have been described with from four to seven
conjugated bonds which impart rigidity to the molecule.   The
carbon chain on the opposing side of the ring contains a large
number of hydroxyl groups creating a flexible hydrophilic region.
Some polyenes additionally contain an amino-sugar moiety.

It has been demonstrated that polyene antibiotics will bind
only to those membranes which contain sterols (Hammond 1977).
Sterols exhibit a restricted distribution in nature being
necessary for the structure and function of eukaryote membranes
but absent from the membranes of prokaryotes.   The incorporation
of sterol into membranes causes the hydrocarbon chains of the
phospholipids to be in an "intermediate fluid condition"; in the
presence of sterols the hydrocarbon chains are in a state of
conformation restriction intermediate to those in the gel
and liquid crystal phases.   For a sterol to bind to phospholipid
and to produce a preferred membrane conformation it must possess
a 3-β-hydroxyl group, and it is believed that this group is
orientated to the membrane surface.   Cholesterol has an almost
universal distribution in mammalian membranes but is replaced by
other sterols, mainly ergosterol, in fungi.

It is believed that when the polyene molecule reaches the
fungal membrane, there is an initial reaction between the drug
and the 3-β-hydroxyl group of the sterol.   The strong affinity
of the hydrophobic polyene chromophore then drags the drug
molecule into the membrane so that the chromophore lies along-
side the sterol ring.   This not only creates instability in the
fungal membrane by reducing the phospholipid-sterol interactions
but also introduces into the membrane the hydrophilic polyol
surface of the antibiotic.   The intrusion of a hydrophilic chain
into the hydrophobic membrane core may be sufficient to destroy
the selective permeability of the membranes.   Alternatively
it has been suggested that sterol-polyene complexes may come
together to form aggregates with the hydrophilic regions of the
drug arranged in the centre creating a water filled pore (Fig. 6)
surrounded by a hydrophobic region (De Kruijft and Demel 1974).

The changes in membrane permeability caused by polyene
antibiotics are more subtle than those elicited by cationic
antiseptics.   Although almost all of the total free potassium
pool of Candida albicans is lost on exposure to low levels of
polyene antibiotic (Hammond et al 1973), leakage of other
cytoplasmic components does not occur.   It has been demonstrated
that the polyene-induced K^+-leakage is closely followed by
inhibition of yeast glycolysis, presumably since potassium ions
are co-factors in at least 3 distinct steps in the glycolytic

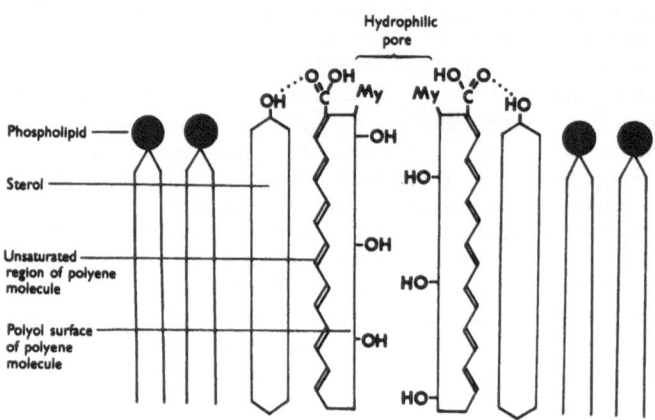

Fig. 6.   Postulated structure of the polyene-sterol pore formed
          in yeast membranes (My = amino sugar, mycosamine).

pathway.   The loss of cations from the cell results in a change
in internal charge and as the membrane has lost its selective
permeability some of the lost cations are replaced (at a pH less
than 7) by protons from the environment.   This results in a
lowering of internal pH and precipitation of cytoplasmic
components (Hammond et al. 1973)

     Polyene antibiotics are used in the control of pathogenic
and opportunistic fungal infections.   Although polyenes have
an affinity for the cholesterol present in mammalian membranes
they possess a somewhat greater avidity for the ergosterol
present in fungal membranes.   This allows sufficient selective
toxicity to permit some polyenes, notably amphotericin B, to be used

intravenously in the treatment of systemic mycoses.   Other polyenes
e.g. nystatin and candicidin, are somewhat less selective and are
used for topical treatment of cutaneous mycoses.

INHIBITORS OF ENERGY TRANSDUCTION BY MICROBIAL MEMBRANES

The energy transducing membranes of mitochondria and bacteria
are able to utilise available substrates to provide energy for the
performance of work, such as the accumulation of metabolites
against a concentration gradient or locomotion.   Two distinct
but inter-related enzyme systems have been implicated in this
phenomena.   The first is the membrane-bound Mg^{2+}-activated
adenosine triphosphatase (Mg^{2+}-ATPase) the terminal enzyme of
oxidative phosphorylation, which catalyses the reaction.

$$ADP + Pi + n\ H^+ \rightleftharpoons ATP + H_2O$$

(where n is pH dependent : 0.7 at pH 7)

The second part involves the enzymes of the electron transport
chain.   Oxidative capacity is not essential for active transport,
since under anaerobic conditions, where organisms have limited
or no oxidative enzyme capacity, active solute uptake may proceed.
Energy-linked transport may also occur in mitrochondrial or
bacterial vesicles made in such a way that ATPase activity cannot
be demonstrated.   This suggests that active transport is not
necessarily coupled directly to ATP hydrolysis and that solute
transport or flagellar motion may be driven by the,'energised
state' of the membrane.   The exact nature of this energised state
is still controversial.   Mitchell in his 'chemiosmotic'
hypothesis suggested a mechanism for the coupling of electron
transfer to ATP synthesis, proposing that the electron transport
chain is arranged in loops across the energy-transducing membrane
and as a result of the transfer of two electrons to water, protons
are expelled (Fig. 7).   The electrogenic expulsion of protons
makes the interior negative with respect to the environment.
The proton gradient so formed represents a store of free energy
since each expelled proton experiences a force, the proton motive
force.   The movement of protons back through the membrane in
response to that force may be used to perform work.   The Mg^{2+}-
activated ATPase couples the diffusion of protons through the
membrane with the synthesis of ATP (Fig. 7), two protons being
required/molecule of ATP synthesized.   The proton gradient may also
be used to power uptake or excretion of metabolites, allowing
the electron transport chain to directly drive active transport
without going through ATP (Mitchell 1974).

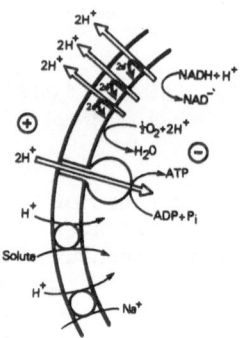

Fig. 7. Chemiosmotic coupling. Electrons and protons from internal
medium are donated to a series of carriers arranged in
loops across the membrane. In mitochondria, there are 3
loops, in bacteria only two. The diffusion of protons
back down the gradient may be coupled to ATP synthesis
or drive solute-uptake using proton symports and solute
excretion by proton antiports.

Energy transduction may be halted by direct inhibition of
the electron transport chain, by the uncoupling of oxidative
phosphorylation from ATP synthesis or by direct inhibition of
the Mg^{2+}-ATPase.

Uncouplers of Oxidative Phosphorylation

In the presence of oxidizable substrate, ADP and inorganic
phosphate the rates of mitochondrial respiration are fast (Fig. 8A)
and the mitochondria are in the active state. In the controlled
state, that is, in the presence of substrate and oxygen but in
the absence of ADP (or phosphate), there is little respiration
in tightly-coupled mitochondria, the rate of respiration being
controlled by the ADP/ATP ratio. When this ratio is high,
respiration is rapid but under conditions where ATP accumulates
at the expense of ADP (i.e. when the rate of energy requirement
falls below the rate of ATP synthesis) respiration rate falls.
This phenomenon, known as respiratory control,is found in
mitochondria, but not in bacteria.

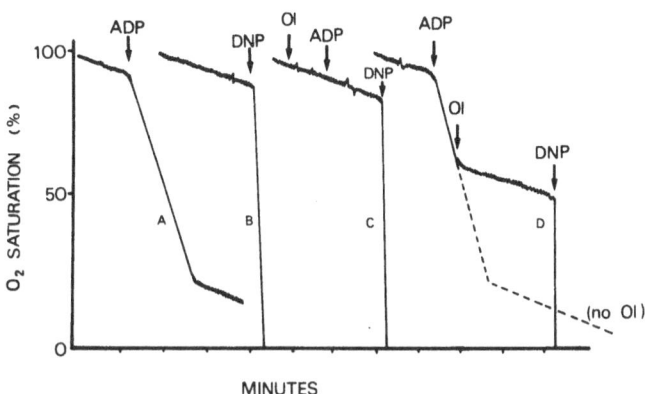

Fig. 8. Comparison of the effects of uncouplers, e.g. DNP and an
inhibitor of Mg^{2+}-ATPase, e.g. oligomycin on the O_2-
consumption of rat liver mitochondria. Oxygen consumption
of freshly prepared mitochondria suspended in buffer
(containing respiratory substrate, P_i and Mg^{2+}). Under
these conditions the mitochondria are tightly coupled so
addition of ADP increases O_2-consumption until all exogenous
ADP is phosphorylated and the O_2-consumption returns to
original level (A). Addition of DNP causes a more marked
stimulation of O_2-consumption (B). In contrast oligomycin
(OL) does not inhibit the respiration rate but blocks the
ADP-stimulation of O_2-consumption (C), however, DNP will
still stimulate O_2 consumption in the presence of oligomycin
(C). Addition of oligomycin also prevents the ADP
stimulation of O_2-uptake (D).

The best known uncouplers include 2, 4-dinitrophenol (DNP),
carbonylcyanide m-chlorophenylhydrazone (CCCP), carbonylcyanide
p-trifluoromethylphenylhydrazone (FCCP) and trichlorosalicylanilide.
DNP and many other uncouplers are weak lipophilic acids able to
dissolve in the hydrophobic interior of the membranes and carry
protons from regions of high to regions of low hydrogen ion
concentration, i.e. effectively short-circuiting the proton
motive force. Uncouplers, by dissipating the 'energised state'
of the membrane, deprive the ATP synthetase of its energy input
thereby halting ATP synthesis. In the presence of uncoupler
respiratory control is lost, allowing substrate utilization to
proceed at maximum rate (Fig. 8A) producing heat rather than
ATP.

Drugs Affecting Mg⁺-activated ATPase

There are great similarities between the membrane bound
ATPase of mitochondria and the equivalent enzymes of chloroplasts
and bacteria. Treatment of mammalian mitochondria with urea
releases a water soluble ATPase, termed F_1, which has been
extensively purified. Purified F_1 is cold labile yielding
five types of protein sub-unit (α - ε), none of which had
enzymic activity. The active site was thought to be located
in the two heaviest sub-units (α and β), since trypsin treatment
yielded a protein containing only these units with intact ATPase
activity.

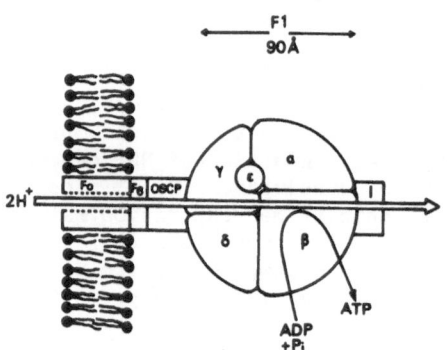

Fig. 9   Proton-translating membrane bound Mg^{2+}-ATPase of
mitochondria. The enzyme consists of 3 regions (a) the
F_1, the ATPase proper, situated in projections coating the
inside of the mitochondrial membrane (b) the F_6/OSCP
region which serves to connect F_1 to the membrane and
(c) the proton-translocating section of the enzyme proteolipid complex (F_0) located in the membrane. Passage of 2
protons through the proton channel facilities the
formation of 1 molecule of ATP from ADP and P_1. The actual
site of synthesis is probably the β-subunit.

Ammonia-treatment released a polypeptide, known as the oligomycin sensitivity-conferring protein (OSCP), which has been shown to be necessary to the binding of F_1 to the membrane. A part of the ATPase known as F_0 is an integral part of the mitochondrial membrane and consists of 3-4 hydrophobic proteins with no discernable ATPase activity. It is believed that F_0 is a proton conducting channel within the membrane, sealed by the binding of F_1. The F_0/F_1 complex of yeast although superficially similar to that of mammalian mitochondria has many significant differences (Hammond 1979).

The membranes of bacteria contain a prominent Mg^{2+}-ATPase, and these complexes have been purified from many bacterial species. The best-studied bacterial ATPase is the Mg^{2+}-activated enzyme from Streptococcus faecalis (Hammond 1979). Electron microscope studies indicate that superficially the enzyme is very similar to that of mitochondria and is located on the inner surface of the cytoplasmic membrane. Differences have been demonstrated in both the composition and sub-unit size in purified soluble ATPase from bacteria (BF_1) and mitochondria (F_1) (Haddock and Jones, 1977). BF_1 proteins are immunologically and functionally distinct from those present in F_1. OSCP is not found in the BF_1/BF_0 complex, the linking function being served by the ε-subunit.

It is possible to divide the true inhibitors of Mg^{2+}-ATPase into two groups. Inhibitors shown to act on both the soluble and the membrane bound ATPase are believed to have their site of action in the F_1 and BF_1 region of the enzyme (Fig. 9). Those agents which only inhibit the enzyme while it is membrane-bound and have no effect upon the purified soluble enzyme and are able to reduce proton permeability of preparations devoid of F_1 or BF_1 have their primary action in the proteolipid region of the membrane i.e. the F_0 or BF_0 (Fig. 10).

Specific binding sites have been ascribed to many of the inhibitors of the ATPase complex. The use of synchronous cultures of the fission yeast Schizosaccharomyces pombe has allowed the temporal resolution of the inhibitor-sensitivity of the ATPase. The inhibitors of the F_0 component can be divided into two groups; site I includes oligomycin, rutamycin venturicidins and alkyltins, while site II includes N^1,N^1dicyclohexylcarbodiimide (DCCD) and leucinostatin. Similarly agents capable of inhibiting the F_1 region can be separated into five other distinct sites i.e. efrapeptin (III), NbfCl (IV), quercitin (VI) and spegazzine (VI) (Lloyd and Edwards, 1977).

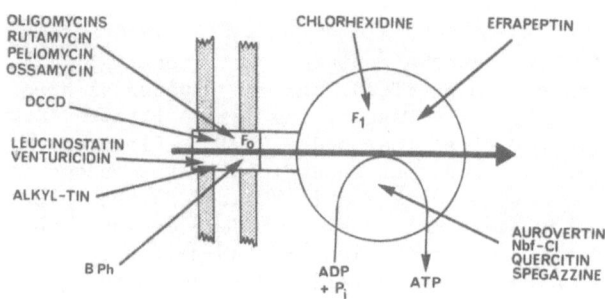

Fig. 10. Inhibitors of bacterial and mitochondrial membrane-
bound Mg^{2+}-ATPase.

Oligomycin is a macrolide antibiotic mixture produced by
a _Streptomyces_ species and is closely related to rutamycin
produced by _Streptomyces rutgenensis_. The drug has little effect
against bacteria and yeasts but is strongly inhibitory to a limited
number of fungal species and has been used in the treatment of
superficial mycoses. Rutamycin and oligomycin do not bind
to, or inhibit F_1, but are potent inhibitors of the membrane-
bound complex. Inhibition of mitochondrial respiration by
oligomycin is completely reversed by uncouplers (see Fig. 8D),

i.e. the drug does not act on the electron transport chain but upon some phase of energy-transfer associated with the terminal step of electron transfer, probably the incorporation of inorganic phosphate into ATP. Oligomycin binds to the oligomycin sensitivity-conferring protein and F_0 in such a way as to prevent translocation through F_0, thereby starving the ATPase of the protons necessary for driving ATP synthesis. Neither purified, nor membrane-bound bacterial ATPase is inhibited by oligomycin. It appears that although $\int$-subunit of the bacterial enzyme is functionally analogous to the OSCP of the mitochondrial enzyme; it cannot bind oligomycin rendering the enzyme insensitive to the drug.

The venturicidins are anti-fungal antibiotics produced by Streptomyces aureofaciens and possess a lactone ring similar to that of oligomycin. The venturicidins have been shown to be more effective in inhibiting the Mg^{2+}-ATPase of yeast mitochondria and that venturicidin acts at a site close to, but distinct from, that of oligomycin. Ossamycin and peliomycin, produced by Streptomyces luteogriseus and hygroscopicus respectively, possess little antibacterial action and some activity against moulds and yeasts. Both are potent inhibitors of the membrane bound enzyme but have little effect upon purified F_1.

Leucinostatin is a polypeptide antibiotic isolated from Penicillium lilacium, which is inactive against Gram-negative bacteria, moderately active against Gram-positive bacteria but very active against a wide range of pathogenic moulds and yeasts. It is believed that leucinostatin binds at a site distinct from oligomycin and the interaction of the drug with the enzyme requires the presence of membrane phospholipid.

A variety of organic agents have also been shown to be potent inhibitors of the F_0 region of the ATPase, including N' N'-dicyclohexylcarbodiimide (DCCD), bathophenanthroline and organic tin compounds. These compounds have been shown to bind to the enzyme at sites other than that used by oligomycin.

Three antibiotics aurovertin, efrapeptin and DIO9, and the well known antiseptic chlorhexidine inhibit the soluble enzyme, i.e. interact directly with F_1 or BF_1.

Aurovertin is produced by Calcarisporium arbuscula and shows little antibacterial activity but some antifungal and anti-protozoal activity. The drug inhibits the soluble ATPase of mitochondria and bacteria. It has been shown that in mammalian and fungal mitochondria the drug binds to the β-subunit of F_1, which is believed to contain the active site of the enzyme.

Efrapeptin, is a polypeptide antibiotic which acts in a way very
similar to aurovertin, but the binding of the two drugs is not
mutually exclusive.   DIO9 is an antibiotic of unknown structure
which inhibits both membrane-bound and soluble Mg^{2+}-ATPase of
fungi and bacteria, halting net K^+-uptake without affecting the
membrane-bound NADH dehydrogenase.

As has been mentioned, chlorhexidine at high concentration
destroys the selective permeability properties of the membrane.
At minimum inhibitory concentrations, however, the drug is a
direct inhibitor of bacterial Mg^{2+}-ATPase, inhibiting net K^+-Na^+
exchange in S. faecalis.   Both membrane-bound and solubilized
Mg^{2+}-ATPase from aerobic and anaerobic bacteria are inhibited.

4-chloro-7-nitrobenzofurazan, quercitin, spegazzine and
acetylguanine have also been shown to interact with the F_1 region
of the membrane-bound ATPase and to inhibit phosphorylation.

Although there are gross differences in the Mg^{2+}-ATPases of
prokaryote and eukaryote none of the agents described have
sufficient selective toxicity to be used in chemotherapy, indeed
most are acutely toxic to mammals.

Inhibitors of the Electron Transport Chain

Reducing equivalents, derived from substrate oxidation, are
transferred to NAD which serves as an intermediary between
catabolite pathways and the components of the cytochrome-chain
which eventually deliver electrons to oxygen to form water.

Streptomyces mobaraensis produces an antibiotic piericidin A,
which has been shown to be an analogue of ubiquinone, an important
component of the electron transport system.   This drug blocks
electron transport at two sites: at very low concentrations it
inhibits oxidation of $NADH_2$ and reduction of ubiquinone, while
at higher concentrations it blocks electron transport between
succinate and ubiquinone, in both mammalian and bacterial cells.
Antimycins, produced by Streptomyces sp. are potent respiratory
inhibitors of eukaryotic cells but have no effect against bacterial
systems.   The antiseptic hexachloraphene has been shown to inhibit
cytochromes and dehydrogenase   enzymes in B. subtilis and
E. coli and to halt respiration in B. megaterium at a site near
the terminal electron acceptor.

AGENTS WHICH DIRECTLY INHIBIT MEMBRANE BIOSYNTHESIS

Although a reduction in membrane biosynthesis is often observed on exposure to antimicrobial agents, there are few examples of compounds which bring about their lethal action by direct inhibition of membrane biosynthesis.

Cerulenin (2, 3 epoxy-4-oxo-7,10 dodecadienoylamide) produced by Cephalosporium caerulens, is inhibitory to the growth of a wide range of bacteria and fungi. It has been shown to be a potent inhibitor of fatty acid biosynthesis, both in vivo and in vitro (Omura, 1976). The drug forms a covalent complex with β-keto acyl ACP-synthase (Fig. 11) thereby depriving the fatty acid biosynthetic pathway of two carbon fragments. In addition cerulenin also halts the synthesis of those macrolides whose synthesis also requires two carbon fragments e.g. flavenoids, macrolide antibiotics, etc. In eukaryotic micro-organisms sterol biosynthesis is prevented by an interaction of cerulenin with 3 hydroxy 3 methylglutaryl-CoA (HMG-CoA) synthetase which is known to be a rate limiting enzyme of overall sterol synthesis. Since cerulenin specifically inhibits HMG-CoA synthesis it is supposed that the action of the drug is distinct from iodocetamide which deactivates both HMG-CoA synthesis and acetoacetyl-CoA-thiolase.

A number of derivatives of diazoborane and boronic acid have been shown to be bacteriostatic towards enteric bacteria (Bailey et al, 1980). These compounds appear to possess a common mechanism of action and mutants resistant to ICI 78911 (a diazoborane derivative) are also resistant to ICI 75188 (a boronic acid). The drugs markedly inhibit the incorporation of acetate into the extractable lipid fraction of E. coli. An examination of the effects of ICI 78911 upon in vitro fatty acid biosynthesis has revealed that the drug acts at a site in the pathway distinct from cerulenin, iodoacetamide and N-ethyl-maleimide, probably upon the acetyl acyl carrier protein transferase (Fig. 11). (Hammond - unpublished observations).

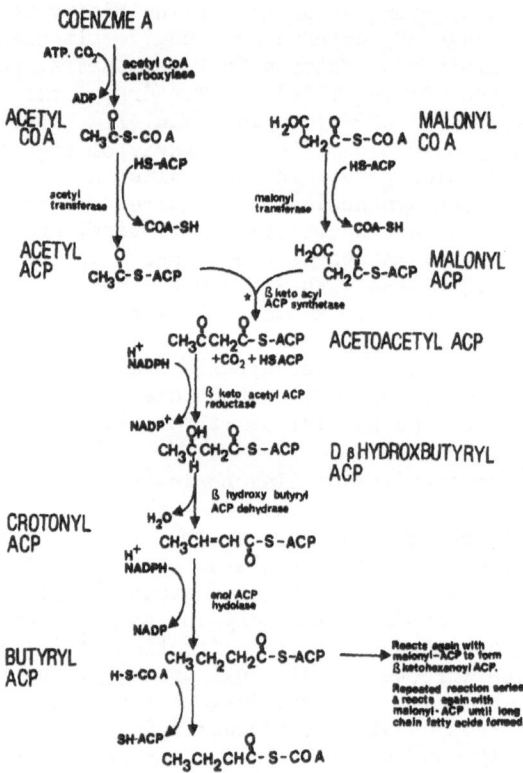

Fig. 11.   Fatty acid biosynthesis in <u>Escherichia coli</u>.

REFERENCES

Bailey, P.J., Cousins, G., Snow, G.A. and White, A.J. (1980).
Boron containing antibacterial agents: effects on growth and
morphology. Antimicrobial Agents and Chemotherapy, 17, 548-553.

De Kruijf, B. and Demel, R.A. (1974). Polyene antibiotic - sterol
interaction in membranes of Acholeoplasma laidlawii and liposomes.
Biochemica et Biophysica Acta. 339, 57-70.

Haddock, B.A. and Jones, C.W. (1977). Bacterial respiration.
Bacteriological Reviews. 41, 47-99.

Hammond, S.M. (1977). Biological activity of polyene antibiotics.
Progress in Medicinal Chemistry. 14, 105-179.

Hammond, S.M. (1979). Inhibitors of enzymes of microbial
membranes: agents affecting Mg^{2+}-activated adenosine
triphosphatase. Progress in Medicinal Chemistry. 16, 223-257.

Hammond, S.M. and Lambert, P.A. (1973). Potassium fluxes: first
indications of membrane damage in micro-organisms. Biochemical
and Biophysical Research Communications. 54, 796-799.

Hammond, S.M., Lambert, P.A. and Kliger, B.N. (1974). The mode of
action of polyene antibiotics; induced potassium leakage in
Candida albicans. Journal of General Microbiology. 81, 325-330.

Hammond, S.M., Lambert, P.A. and Kliger, B.N. (1974). The mode
of action of polyene antibiotics: induced entry of hydrogen ions
in Candida albicans. Journal of General Microbiology. 81,
331-336.

Harold, P.M., Baarda, J.R., Baron, C. and Abrahams, A. (1969).
DIO9 and chlorhexidine: inhibitors of membrane-bound ATPase and
of cation transport in S. faecalis. Biochemica et Biophysica
Acta. 183, 129-136.

Helenius, A. and Simons, K. (1975). Solubilization of membranes
by detergents. Biochemica et Biophysica Acta. 415, 29-79.

Hugo, W.B. (1971). Inhibition and Distruction of the Microbial
Cell. Academic Press, London.

Lambert, P.A. (1978). Membrane-active antimicrobial agents.
Progress in Medicinal Chemistry. 15, 87-124.

Lloyd, D. and Edwards, S.W. (1976). Mitochondrial ATPase of the fission yeast Schizosaccharomyces pombe. Biochemical Journal. 160, 335-342.

Mitchell, P. (1974). A chemiosmotic molecular mechanism for proton-translocating ATPase. FEBS Letters. 43, 189-194.

Omura, S. (1976). The antibiotic cerulenin. Bacteriological Reviews. 40, 681-697.

Russell, A.D., Morris, A. and Allwood, M.C. (1973). in Methods in Microbiology. 8, eds. J.R. Norris and D.W. Ribbons. Academic Press, London p.95.

Simoni, R.D. and Postma, P.W. (1975). The energetics of bacterial active transport. Annual Review of Biochemistry. 44, 523-554.

Smith, A.R.W., Lambert, P.A., Hammond, S.M. and Jessup, C. (1975). Differing effects of cetyltrimethylammonium bromide and cetrimide BP upon growing cultures of E. coli. Journal of Applied Bacteriology. 38, 143-149.

Antibiotics affecting microbial cell walls: Progress after 112 years

Professor S Selwyn

Department of Medical Microbiology
Westminster Medical School, Horseferry Road
London, SW1P 2AR, UK

ANTIBIOTICS OTHER THAN BETA-LACTAM COMPOUNDS

Although the beta-lactam antibiotics are by the far the most important therapeutic agents that act by inhibiting bacterial cell-wall peptidoglycan synthesis, several other totally unrelated antibiotics act at earlier stages of this essential pathway (Selwyn, 1980a). The clinically significant members of this miscellaneous group of drugs are bacitracin, vancomycin, cycloserine and phosphomycin. Others of less importance include novobiocin and ristocetin. The current position in relation to each can be briefly reviewed.

Bacitracin

This bactericidal antibiotic was originally isolated from *Bacillus subtilis* as long ago as 1945. It consists of a mixture of related polypeptides, which, interestingly, contain a thiazolidine ring as does penicillin. Bacitracin inhibits the regeneration of phospholipid carriers required for the incorporation of pentaglycine and N-acetylglucosamine in the developing peptidoglycan molecule.

In spite of a high risk of nephrotoxicity, bacitracin was for many years administered by injection in short courses to treat otherwise resistant staphylococcal infections. This is now no longer justified, and the antibiotic is used only topically; in combination with antibiotics such as the polymyxins or neomycin to supplement its activity (which is limited to Gram-positive bacteria) bacitracin remains one of the main agents used locally in skin infections (Selwyn, 1981). It is also still the most convenient indicator in primary cultures of *Streptococcus pyogenes* belonging to Lancefield Group A.

Vancomycin

Originally isolated in 1955 from *Streptomyces orientalis*, vancomycin is a bactericidal antibiotic which inhibits peptidoglycan synthesis (at one stage later than bacitracin) apparently by forming complexes with essential peptide components. Although ototoxicity, nephrotoxicity and tissue irritation are hazards of therapy, intravenous administration remains of value in serious Gram-positive infections where safer antibiotics cannot be used due to resistance or allergy. In particular, vancomycin is a reserve drug for severe *Staphylococcus aureus* or *Staphylococcus epidermidis* infections.

Recently another important use has emerged - in pseudomembranous colitis, which is usually a complication of antibiotic therapy due to the encouragement of bowel overgrowth with toxigenic *Clostridium difficile*. Oral vancomycin has proved highly effective in this extremely dangerous condition. This and other aspects of vancomycin therapy have recently been reviewed by Brown and Wise (1982).

Cycloserine

This was also first isolated in 1955, from *Streptomyces garyphalus*, and is a derivative of D-serine with a relatively simple molecule (D-4-amino-3-isoxazolidone), which as in the case of chloramphenicol can be readily synthesised. It is a D-alanine analogue which acts at one of the earliest stages of cell wall synthesis by inhibiting alanine racemase and so preventing the incorporation of D-alanine into the pentapeptide component of peptidoglycan. It has a relatively broad spectrum of action against Gram positive and Gram-negative bacteria.

Cycloserine has the advantage of being absorbed by mouth but often produces neurological side effects. It remains a reserve drug for the treatment of tuberculosis in combination with other agents. It has also been used for the treatment of urinary tract infections (Garrod *et al.*, 1981) but this now no longer seems justifiable.

Phosphomycin' (Fosfomycin, Phosphonomycin)

This antibiotic was isolated in 1969 from *Streptomyces fradii*, and like cycloserine has a very simple structure with a molecular weight of 102. It is an analogue of p-enolpyruvate, which also inhibits one of the earliest stages of cell wall synthesis - the activation of phosphoenolpyruvate, and its subsequent incorporation into the uridinedinucleotide-N-acetylmuramic acid complex.

The antibiotic has a relatively broad spectrum, and it has been reported to be safe and effective in a wide range of infections. Its use has so far been mainly restricted to Spanish hospitals (Symposium, 1977), and the results of further studies are awaited.

Miscellaneous Antibiotics

Novobiocin is another antibiotic that was first isolated in 1955 - from *Streptomyces spheroides*. Although it appears to have an inhibitory effect on the early stages of cell wall synthesis this may be secondary to its other activities, which include inhibition of DNA polymerase and both RNA synthesis and degradation. The cell membrane is also damaged in some bacteria. These effects are exerted mainly on Gram-positive bacteria, and novobiocin has for many years been held in reserve for the oral treatment of staphylococcal infections. However, because of its interference with liver function, its high protein binding and other drawbacks, a case can be made for abandoning the use of novobiocin (Garrod *et al.*, 1981).

Ristocetin which was originally isolated in 1957 from *Nocardia lurida* has also been regarded as a reserve drug for use in staphylococcal infections and in some difficult infections due to non-haemolytic streptococci. One of its activities is said to be the inhibition of an early stage of cell wall synthesis. As with the similar antibiotic, vancomycin, ristocetin acts only on Gram-positive bacteria (Barker and Prescott, 1973).

Other Alanine Analogues. Several of these have been investigated in recent years. One of the most promising appears to be S-alanyl-R-1-amino-ethylphosphoric acid (Ro 03-7008) which acts in a similar way to cycloserine by preventing D-alanine incorporation into peptidoglycan. Little has been heard of this compound since a preliminary review (Editorial, 1978).

PENICILLINS

Crude preparations and extracts of moulds have been used in folk medicine both topically and orally for many centuries. However, the first scientific observations on the antibacterial effects of *Penicillium* species took place not - as is generally believed - in 1928-29, with the celebrated work of Alexander Fleming, but almost 60 years earlier between 1870 and 1876 in several British laboratories - notably that of Joseph Lister in Edinburgh (Selwyn, 1979a). Some equally fascinating recent historical researches have radically altered our picture of the circumstances and interpretation of Fleming's famous observations, and have modified the popular account of the definitive work carried out on penicillin in Oxford from 1938 until 1942 by Howard Florey, Ernst Chain and their colleagues (Selwyn, 1980b).

After the widespread introduction of benzylpenicillin at the end of World War II the only piece of material progress before 1960 was the realisation that phenoxymethyl penicillin (originally produced in 1948) was relatively well absorbed by mouth. It was subsequently introduced in 1954 as 'penicillin V.' This was three years before the really important advance took place at the Beecham Research Laboratories in Surrey, England. Here under the guidance of Ernst Chain, George Rolinson and his colleagues isolated the penicillin 'nucleus' (6-amino-penicillanic acid or 6-APA). This consists of a fused beta-lactam ring and a thiazolidine ring, in which the latter has two methyl groups inserted at the 2-carbon, and a carboxyl at the 3-carbon; the four-membered beta-lactam ring has, apart from the essential oxygen at the 7-carbon, an amino group at the 6-carbon. It was now at last possible to produce versatile derivatives semi-synthetically by the insertion of a wide range of side chains at the 6-carbon position of the all-important beta-lactam ring.

'Penicillinase-resistant' Penicillins

The first practical result of the Beecham work was the introduction in 1960 of methicillin (2,2-dimethoxyphenyl-penicillin). This antibiotic, which is given by injection, was able to withstand the beta-lactamase or 'penicillinase' enzyme produced by *Staph. aureus* which rapidly hydrolyses penicillin and irreversibly opens up the beta-lactam ring. The presence of a 'bulky' side chain at the 6-carbon evidently exerts 'steric

hindrance' to the attachment of staphylococcal beta-lactamase
(but, curiously, not usually to the enzymes from other bacteria).
In 1961, the orally available derivative cloxacillin, which has
similar resistance to the staphylococcal enzyme, was introduced
as the first member of the isoxazolyl penicillins, which include
oxacillin and dicloxacillin. These all have the pharmacokinetic
defect of very high binding (c.95%) to human serum albumin.
Protein binding is not a significant problem with other
penicillins, although it is with some cephalosporins such as
cefazolin, as discussed later.

After the introduction of flucloxacillin in 1970 (on the
controversial basis of allegedly better absorption from the
intestine) there have been no further developments in this group
of penicillins, which remain one of the standard treatments for
staphylococcal infections. Nafcillin, a naphthamido analogue of
methicillin introduced about 20 years ago outside the U.K.
requires to be mentioned in this context. Although it is very
stable to staphylococcal beta-lactamase, it is erratically absorbed
by mouth and is eliminated largely by biliary excretion and
metabolic inactivation, renal excretion accounting for an
unusually low 10% or so.

Ampicillin and Related 'Broad-spectrum' Penicillins

In 1961, one year after the introduction of methicillin, the
insertion of an amino group at the α-position of the benzylpenicillin side chain gave rise to ampicillin - a penicillin
whose activity extended to many Gram-negative bacteria, such as
typhoid bacilli and *Haemophilus influenzae* (the penicillin
resistance of which formed the basis of Fleming's classic 1929
paper). Ampicillin and its derivatives unfortunately possess no
enhanced resistance to most beta-lactamases and they have indeed
generally decreased potency compared with benzylpenicillin against
Gram-positive bacteria (except faecal streptococci) and neisseriae.

Ampicillin is correctly regarded as the first 'broad-spectrum'
penicillin, but it was not the first penicillin to show activity
against Gram-negative bacilli. Such an antibiotic had been
available in crude form since 1945 following the isolation of the
Sardinian mould which eventually gave rise to the cephalosporin N,
later renamed penicillin N (D-4-amino-4-carboxy-n-butylpenicillin),
which was purified in Oxford in 1949 (Selwyn, 1982). Although
found to be useful in typhoid as 'adicillin' this antibiotic was
never produced commercially.

Ampicillin Analogues. The next major development in
the broad-spectrum penicillins was the introduction in 1967 of
carbenicillin; but this is not a close analogue of ampicillin and
is therefore included in the subsequent section. The true analogue
of ampicillin, amoxycillin (amoxicillin in the U.S.A.) was
produced in 1972 by simply inserting an hydroxyl group at the
para position in the benzyl side chain of ampicillin. This
resulted in an improvement in intestinal absorption from
approximately 30% for ampicillin to about 70% for amoxycillin.
In addition, bacterial killing *in vitro* is more rapid with
amoxycillin, as discussed in a later section; this is also the
case with the ampicillin analogue, epicillin which contains a
cyclohexadien group instead of a benzene ring in the side chain.
Epicillin was introduced in 1972 - the same year as amoxycillin -
but not in the U.K.

Two earlier analogues to be noted are ciclacillin and
hetacillin, both dating from 1965. Ciclacillin (or cyclacillin in
the U.S.A.), introduced in the U.K. in 1980, contains a complicated
sounding group in the side chain (1-aminocyclohexanecarboxamido-).
Although it is as well absorbed as amoxycillin, its antibacterial
activity appears to be significantly lower than that of ampicillin.

Hetacillin, which is not available in the U.K., was initially
regarded as a separate antibiotic from ampicillin. In fact, despite
a complex side chain it is hydrolysed in the body to ampicillin
and acetone. It may therefore be regarded as a 'pro-drug' of
ampicillin, like the esters which are now to be described.

Ampicillin Esters. Intestinal absorption of ampicillin
has been more than doubled in several cases by esterification.
Free ampicillin is released during and immediately after
absorption of each pro-drug. Pivampicillin was first described
in 1970 but was not made available in the U.K. until 1980.
Talampicillin (a phthalidyl ester) was introduced in 1974, and
bacampicillin in 1980. In addition to better uptake from an oral
dose, less intestinal disturbance than with ampicillin has been
claimed for these esters - but to offset this, more upper gastrointestinal irritation has been observed in some studies.

The activity of the ampicillin group has recently been
extended by administering amoxycillin in combination with the
beta-lactamase inhibitor, clavulanic acid. This potentially
important advance is discussed in a later section. The ureido-
penicillins, mezlocillin and azlocillin, as well as piperacillin
may be regarded as ampicillin analogues, but they can be

conveniently discussed with the other anti-pseudomonal penicillins in the next section.

Anti-pseudomonal Penicillins

The introduction of carbenicillin(α-carboxybenzylpenicillin) in 1967 provided for the first time activity against *Pseudomonas aeruginosa,* but with a further loss of potency against most organisms sensitive to ampicillin. The antibiotic has to be injected and large doses are required due to relatively high minimum inhibitory concentrations (MICs). As the disodium salt is used this entails the administrations of large doses of sodium ions, causing a potential problem of overloading. Carbenicillin has usually been used as an adjunct to aminoglycoside therapy.

In 1974, an orally absorbed ester of carbenicillin - carfecillin - became available; but its use seems justifiable only in the uncommon urinary tract infections due to pseudomonads or certain other problematical Gram-negative bacilli. A slight increase in the activity of carbenicillin was achieved when in 1979 ticarcillin (the 3-thienylmethyl analogue) was introduced in the U.K.

More significant progress was marked by the development of acyl-ureido derivatives of penicillin, which were introduced in the U.K. in 1980. Azlocillin possesses up to eight times as much anti-pseudomonal activity as carbenicillin. Greater activity against Enterobacteriaceae members but less against pseudomonads is shown by the close analogue, mezlocillin (which possesses a terminal methyl-sulphonyl group in place of the hydrogen atom of azlocillin). However, the related piperazine-aminobenzylpenicillin derivative, piperacillin, combines the best features of each antibiotic, and has indeed a potency against pseudomonads and many other Gram-negative bacilli which is comparable to that of gentamicin (Selwyn, 1982). All three antibiotics tend to have a synergistic action with gentamicin and newer aminoglycosides. Moreover, because of the lower dosage requirements and presence of less sodium in their salts, the three new derivatives have minimal risk of sodium and water overloading compared with carbenicillin or ticarcillin. None of the penicillins in this group possesses resistance to beta-lactamases other than those commonly produced by pseudomonads.

A summary of the comparative features of broad spectrum penicillins is given in Table I.

53

TABLE I.   Comparison of the major penicillins

	Routes given	β-lact. stable[1]	Low Sodium	Active against[2] Gram+	Gram-	Pseud.	Ano[2]
Penicillin G	Injection	-	++	++++[3]	-[4]	-	++
Penicillin V	Oral	-	++[5]	+++	-	-	+
Cloxacillin grp.	Oral/Inj.	+++[6]	-	++[6]	-	-	-
Ampicillin grp.	Oral/Inj.	-	++	++[7]	++	-	++
'Augmentin'	Oral/Inj.	+++	++[5]	+++[7]	(++++)	-	++
Carbenicillin	Oral/Inj.	-	-	+	++	+	+
Ticarcillin	Inj.	-	+	+	++	++	+
Mezlocillin	Inj.	-	+++	+	+++	++	+++
Azlocillin	Inj.	-	+++	+	++	+++	++
Piperacillin	Inj.	-	+++	++[7]	+++[8]	++++	+++
Mecillinam	Oral/Inj.	-	++	-[9]	++[10]	-	-
Temocillin	Inj.	+++	+	-	+++	-	-

'-' to '+++' indicates increasingly satisfactory properties. [1]Stability to β-lactamases.
[2]Gram-positive and Gram-negative bacteria, pseudomonads and anaerobes, respectively.
[3]Excludes Strep. faecalis and many Staph. aureus. [4]Excludes neisseriae.
[5]Potassium orally. [6]Chiefly Staph. aureus. [7]Includes Strep. faecalis. [8]Includes H. influenzae.
[9]Excludes urinary staphylococci. [10]Urinary only.

Amidino-penicillins and Temocillin

Mecillinam. In place of the customary attachment of the penicillin side chain by means of an amino group (R-CO-NH-), an amidino group (R-CH=N-) can serve. At present, mecillinam remains the only available amidino-penicillin. It was first described in 1972 and later introduced for oral use esterified as the pivaloyl form (analogous to pivampicillin), and subsequently was made available as an injection of the unmodified antibiotic. Its use is virtually restricted to Gram-negative urinary tract infections, due to its limited spectrum of activity and the poor tissue concentrations achieved. Mecillinam possesses minimal resistance to most beta-lactamases.

Temocillin. This interesting new antibiotic designated disodium 6β-(2-carboxy-2-thiem-3-yl-acetamido)6α-methoxy-penicillanate, has a methoxy group inserted at the 6α-position of the penicillin nucleus which is analogous to the substituent in cefoxitin, as described later. The resulting molecule in each case is highly resistant to beta-lactamases. In fact, temocillin is the first clinically useful penicillin to possess a combination of good activity against Gram-negative bacilli and resistance to beta-lactamases. However, it has no significant activity against pseudomonads, *Bacteroides fragilis* or Gram-positive bacteria (Slocombe *et al.*, 1981). Reports on clinical trials are now awaited.

CEPHALOSPORINS

The isolation of cephalosporin C in 1955 by Edward Abraham and Guy Newton at Oxford occurred just 10 years after the discovery of the original *Cephalosporium acremonium* mould by Guiseppe Brotzu from a sewage outfall on the beach at Cagliari, Sardinia (Selwyn, 1980b). Although cephalosporin C has good resistance to various beta-lactamases, it has relatively poor antibacterial activity. Fortunately, in 1960 the source of numerous more useful cephalosporins was produced in adequate amounts. This was the 7-amino-cephalosporanic acid (7-ACA) nucleus, which is closely similar to that of penicillin, except for the fusion of the beta-lactam ring to a six-membered dihydrothiazine ring rather than a five-membered thiazolidine ring.

55

'First Generation' Cephalosporins

By 1964, two cephalosporins had been introduced into clinical practice - cephaloridine from Glaxo Laboratories in the U.K. and cephalothin from Eli Lilly Laboratories in the U.S.A. Both required to be injected; but in 1967 an oral derivative cephalexin was introduced, followed in 1972 by a further injectable variety, cefazolin (or cephazolin), and an analogue of cephalexin that could be given orally or parenterally - cephradine. At the same time two analogues of cephalothin - cephapirin and cephacetrile - were made available abroad. Five years later another oral analogue of cephalexin, cefadroxil, was also introduced outside the U.K.

The first five of the cephalosporins, which were available in the U.K., were compared by means of detailed *in vitro* and *in vivo* tests (Selwyn, 1976). Cephaloridine (which is the most nephrotoxic - followed by cephalothin) was, together with cefazolin, shown to be the least resistant to beta-lactamases. Cephalexin was more resistant to beta-lactamases, and cephradine was found to be the most resistant. Cephradine also performed best in the animal protection tests despite relatively high MICs in conventional tests on the bacterial strains used. A similar divergence between good clinical results and mediocre laboratory findings has been observed with cephradine in serious infections such as staphylococcal endocarditis. Its favourable pharmaco-kinetic properties coupled with its resistance to common beta-lactamases are important factors underlying such discrepancies.

Cephalothin performed the poorest in the experimental animal infections, and this is in keeping with the need to administer cephalothin in relatively large doses, which are painful and have a particular tendency to produce thrombophlebitis when given intravenously.

In subsequent tests, cephapirin, cephacetrile and cefadroxil were found to possess no advantages over the equivalent analogues available in the U.K.

'Second Generation' Cephalosporins

First described between 1973 and 1976, cefoxitin, cefamandole (cephamandole) and cefuroxime were introduced into the U.K. in 1978. In addition a new oral derivative of cephalexin, cefaclor, was introduced in 1979.

Cefoxitin is not a true cephalosporin but is correctly called a 'cephamycin' since it is derived from *Streptomyces lactamdurans* and not from the original mould via 7-ACA. Like temocillin, cefoxitin has a methoxy group inserted in the α-position at the origin of the side chain on the beta-lactam ring. This appears to be the basis of the resistance to beta-lactamases of both drugs. Cefoxitin unfortunately has poorer activity than the first generation cephalosporins against Gram-positive bacteria; it also has relatively unfavourable pharmacokinetics and frequently causes thrombophlebitis. Its use seemed originally justified for problematical Gram-negative and anaerobic infections, but cefuroxime or the newer derivative cefotaxime (discussed later) is preferable for the former, and metronidazole for the latter.

Cefuroxime possesses a methoxime group in its side chain, and this seems to exert considerable steric hindrance to beta-lactamases, but slightly less than the methoxy group of cefoxitin. Cefuroxime is in other respects a more satisfactory antibiotic and is useful as a reserve drug in infections due to beta-lactamase-producing Gram-negative bacteria, including gonococci. An ester for oral use is currently under trial.

In contrast, cefamandole has proved to be disappointing. Initial claims that it possessed considerable resistance to beta-lactamases and other advantages have been refuted (Selwyn, 1980c, 1980d). Similar disappointment was experienced with cefaclor, the cephalexin derivative with a chlorine atom instead of a methyl group at the 3-carbon position. This drug is absorbed less well from the intestine than either cephalexin or cephradine, and it is also less stable to beta-lactamase attack and spontaneous inactivation.

In our own hospital practice, cephradine has for six years remained the 'routine' cephalosporin for oral and parenteral use. However, a small group of newer derivatives, discussed below, is kept in reserve for resistant infections.

'Third Generation' Cephalosporins

These are the latest developments after more than 30 years of research. The aims have been to achieve optimal pharmaco-kinetics and penetration of the bacterial cell wall (a particular problem in many Gram-negative bacilli, notably pseudomonads), high resistance to beta-lactamases, and high affinity of the antibiotic for the major enzymes involved in cell wall synthesis. The ideal combination of these properties has yet to be achieved in practice, and indeed most new derivatives have lost some of the good features of the earlier products. Mention must now be made of cefotaxime, ceftazidime, cefsulodin, cefoperazone and the cephalosporin analogue moxalactam. All possess. for the first time in the cephalosporins, anti-pseudomonal activity - although this is relatively small with cefotaxime. Resistance to beta-lactamases is also of a generally high order, especially with the first two and last antibiotics.

Cefotaxime, produced by Roussel and Hoechst Laboratories, was introduced into the U.K. in 1981, as an injectable drug only. It has proved to be very useful in severe infections due to a wide range of Gram-negative bacilli resistant to other beta-lactam antibiotics, but it has relatively poor activity against Gram-positive bacteria (Selwyn, 1980c). Like cephalothin, cephapirin and cephacetrile, cefotaxime is partially inactivated by de-acetylation, and, among its less favourable pharmacokinetic features, it achieves comparatively low urinary concentrations.

Ceftazidime produced by Glaxo Laboratories, is due to be marketed in the U.K. in 1983, but has been used widely in clinical trials for over a year. It posesses considerably greater anti-pseudomonal activity than other beta-lactam antibiotics except piperacillin and cefsulodin - but even these two drugs are usually somewhat less active than ceftazidime. Once again, high activity against most Gram-negative bacteria is accompanied by relatively poor potency against Gram-positive organisms and bacteroides (Davies, 1982).

This dissociation is seen to an extreme degree with cefsulodin, a derivative produced by Ciba Laboratories which was first marketed in the U.K. in 1982. This antibiotic has some activity only against staphylococci and group A streptococci apart from its anti-pseudomonal activity (Davies, 1982).

Cefoperazone is another new cephalosporin which has attracted considerable attention. However, it seems to possess few interesting features apart from good activity against pseudomonads (Davies, 1982).

Although moxalactam has very similar properties to ceftazidime it is more logically considered with other unusual beta-lactam compounds after the next section. In Table II the major features of the principal cephalosporins are summarised.

Beta-lactamase Inhibitors

Despite claims that cloxacillin or flucloxacillin could

TABLE II.   Comparison of the major cephalosporins*

	Routes given	β-lact. stable[1]	Safety	Free drug[2]	Metab. stable[2]	Pharma-cokinet.[4]	Activity[5]
Cephaloridine	Injection	+	+	+++	++++	+++	-
Cephalothin	Inj.	++	++	++	++	++	6
Cephalexin	Oral	+++	++++	++++	++++	+++	-
Cephradine	Oral/Inj.	++++[7]	++++	++++	++++	++++	8
Cefaclor	Oral	++	++++	++++	++	++	-
Cefazolin	Inj.	+	++++	+	++++	+	-
Cefamandole	Inj.	++[7]	++++[7]	++	++++	++	-
Cefuroxime	Inj.	++++	++++	+++	++++	+++	-
Cefoxitin	Inj.	++++	+++	++	++++	++	8,9
Cefotaxime	Inj.	++++	(++++)	+++	++	+++	9,10
Ceftazidime	Inj.	++++	(++++)	+++	++++	+++	9,10
Cefoperazone	Inj.	++	(++++)	+++	++++	+++	9,10
Cefsulodin	Inj.	++	(++++)	+++	++++	+++	9,10,11
Moxalactam	Inj.	++++	(++++)	+++	++++	+++	9,10

*Cefoxitin (a cephamycin) and moxalactam (a 1-oxacephem) are included for convenience.
'+' to '++++' indicates increasingly satisfactory properties. Parentheses indicate early experience.

[1]Stability to β-lactamases. [2]Relative proportion unbound to body albumin   [3]Resistance to metabolic inactivation. [4]Pharmacokinetic properties. [5]Notes on specific aspects. [6]Relatively large dose needed. [7]With significant exceptions. [8]Very active against anaerobes. [9]Relatively poor activity against Gram-positive bacteria. [10]Anti-pseudomonal activity. [11]Unusually narrow spectrum.

produce useful inhibition of beta-lactamases from Gram-negative bacteria, and so protect ampicillin in combined formulations, these had minimal practical value (Selwyn, 1980c). The isolation of clavulanic and olivanic acids by Beecham Laboratories several years ago provided the first powerful enzyme inhibitors.

Clavulanic Acid This was first reported in 1976 as a product of *Streptomyces clavuligerus*. It contains an oxazolidine instead of a thiazolidine ring fused to a beta-lactam ring, and possesses only weak antibacterial activity, but it is a powerful inhibitor of most beta-lactamases, except some in Class I ('cephalosporinases'). Synergistic action is produced in combination with vulnerable beta-lactam agents against a wide range of enzyme-producing Gram-positive and Gram-negative bacteria (Brown, 1981). Clavulanic acid was first marketed in the U.K. in 1981 as a capsule containing 125 mg combined with 250 mg of amoxycillin under the proprietary name of Augmentin. Clinical results with these capsules and with the more recently introduced parenteral formulation have been generally satisfactory.

Olivanic Acids. These were originally isolated in 1976 from *Streptomyces olivaceus*, and contain a carbon atom instead of the sulphur of penicillin or oxygen of clavulanic acid. In general the olivanic acids have significant antibacterial activity as well as good beta-lactamase inhibitory potency (Brown, 1981).

Thienamycin is closely similar in structure. Originally reported in 1978 from Merck Laboratories as a product of *Streptomyces cattleya*, it has a remarkably broad range of antibacterial activity against most Gram-positive and Gram-negative species, including pseudomonads. Because of instability of the original antibiotic, an N-formimidoyl derivative has been prepared, and is giving very promising results (Selwyn, 1982).

Penicillanic Acid Sulphones. In 1978, Pfizer Laboratories reported the irreversible inhibiting effect on beta-lactamases of CP-45, 899, a synthetic derivative of penicillin with only slight antibacterial activity of its own. Its synergistic effect on other beta-lactam antibiotics seems less pronounced than with clavulanic acid (Brown, 1981).

Other Novel Beta-lactam Antibiotics

The energetic efforts of organic chemists to produce a remarkable range of penem and cephem derivatives have been rivalled by the production of novel beta-lactam compounds - some of which were reviewed in the previous section. Mention in particular may be made of moxalactam and the monocyclic beta-lactams.

Moxalactam (6059S, LY127935). This synthetic derivative of benzylpenicillin possesses a remarkable mixture of features of the leading penicillins and cephalosporins (Brown, 1981): for example, the general structure of a cephalosporin with the sulphur replaced by an oxygen atom; the 7 α-methoxy group of cefoxitin; the para-hydroxybenzyl group of amoxycillin; and the α-carboxyl group of carbenicillin. Laboratory and clinical results with moxalactam are comparable to those with ceftazidime (Davies, 1982), and it is expected that this interesting antibiotic will be marketed in the U.K. before the end of 1982.

Nocardicins. These were originally reported from the Fujisawa Company, Japan in 1976 as products of a *Nocardia* species. They are monocyclic beta-lactams which generally resemble the more conventional fused compounds in their properties. Nocardicin A is the most active so far, with effects limited to Gram-negative species and with good resistance to beta-lactamases (Brown, 1981). The antibiotic is unusual in possessing better activity *in vivo* than *in vitro*, being assisted by the presence of polymorphonuclear leukocytes and perhaps other components of the body.

Monobactams. Relatively simple monocyclic beta-lactam rings were reported in 1981 to have been isolated by the Squibb Company from various bacteria including a very unusual source for a beta-lactam compound - *Chromobacterium violaceum*, rather than a mould or an actinomycete. The molecules contain a sulphonate group attached directly to the nitrogen atom of the beta-lactam ring. Chemical variants of the molecule are easier to obtain, however, by starting with 6-APA. Produced by this route the first example to be submitted to clinical trials - azthreonam (SQ 26,776) - has recently been described in detail (Sykes and Phillips, 1981). This compound has good activity against Gram-negative bacteria, excluding pseudomonads, and good resistance to beta-lactamases. By further modifying the molecule, the spectrum of action can, it is anticipated, be 'tailored' very precisely against any particular bacteria.

PROGRESS ON FUNDAMENTAL ASPECTS

Inhibition of Cell Wall Synthesis

After more than 40 years of research into the mode of action of penicillins and cephalosporins, a reasonably coherent and

61

convincing picture has been built up in recent years (Selwyn, 1980a). The antibiotics inhibit the late stage of cell wall synthesis which involves transpeptidation to form adequate cross linkages in the peptidoglycan polymer. The CO-N bond of the beta-lactam ring apparently competes with the CO-N bond of the D-alanyl-D-alanine in the emerging peptidoglycan for the active site of transpeptidase enzyme. The killing effect of the antibiotics is not only due to simple osmotic damage sustained by bacterial cells which lack adequately protective cell wall peptidoglycan; in addition, there is an uncontrolled action of autolytic endopeptidases which normally work in harmony with the synthetic enzymes to allow the insertion of newly formed portions of peptidoglycan. A deficiency of the autolytic enzymes has been invoked to explain antibiotic 'tolerance' in some staphylococci. Here the bacteria are inhibited at low drug concentrations, but killing does not occur even at very high drug levels.

Penicillin-binding Proteins

In the past 5 years, insight has been gained into the varying abilities of different beta-lactam antibiotics to bind to the synthetic enzymes located on or near the bacterial cell membrane. These are called 'penicillin-binding proteins' (PBPs) in isolated cell membrane preparations, which are treated with 14C-labelled radioactive antibiotics. For example, in *Escherichia coli*, benzylpenicillin binds strongly to PBPs numbered 1A, 1B, 3, 4, 5 and 6, - but only weakly to PBP 2. Mecillinam binds only to PBP 2. Ampicillin and cefuroxime bind mainly to PBP3. These affinities correlate well with the morphological changes which are characteristic of the various antibiotics (Selwyn, 1980a). PBP 3 appears to be responsible mainly for cross-wall trans-peptidation at the time of cell division; ampicillin therefore tends to favour the production of long filamentous bacteria which may remain viable for lengthy periods. Antibiotics, including amoxycillin, which act mainly on PBP 1B and related enzymes have a more widespread effect on cell wall synthesis; this favours the production of spheroplasts, which are highly vulnerable to osmotic damage. This effect is generally correlated with a more rapid bactericidal action *in vitro*. In contrast, PBP 2 seems to have a very localised function at the corners of cells; mecillinam consequently produces osmotically stable ovoid cells. The combination of antibiotics with different affinities may produce synergistic effects; these are reported between mecillinam and, for example, ampicillin.

Other Investigations

Mention may be made of recent work on the effects of sub-inhibitory concentrations of antibiotics, which may facilitate the action of the body's defences. There is current interest also in the concept of 'pulse dosage' regimens based on the need for bacterial growth and multiplication to be present if beta-lactam antibiotics are to achieve a cidal effect. Other important themes of continuing research include the significance of beta-lactamases in resistance to antibiotics, plasmids and transfer of resistance, and structure-activity relationships of beta-lactam antibiotics. These have been reviewed recently (Selwyn, 1980a, 1980d).

CONCLUDING REMARKS

The penicillins and cephalosporins are understandably the most widely used of antibiotics because of their remarkable safety and efficacy. Astonishing progress has been made, particularly, in the past decade, to develop semi-synthetically a vast and possibly bewildering collection of antibiotics, either for specific infections or to cope with an extremely broad range of pathogenic bacteria. Unfortunately, however, every new derivative which has been introduced has important deficiencies to accompany its special virtues. For this reason, discretion and a critical approach is required in the clinicians who use antibiotics and in their laboratory-based colleagues who advise them. Particularly with the numerous beta-lactam agents, rigorous evaluation on a strictly comparative basis must form the foundation of rational antibiotic usage and of the policies and strategies which are intended to be of assistance (Selwyn, 1979c, 1980e).

REFERENCES

Barker, B.M. and Prescott, F. (1973). Antimicrobial Agents in Medicine. Blackwell, Oxford.

Brown, A.G. (1981). New Naturally Occurring β-lactam Antibiotics and Related Compounds. J. antimicrob. Chemother., 7, 15-48.

Brown, R. and Wise, R. (1982). Vancomycin: a Reappraisal. Br. med. J., 284, 1508-1509.

Davies, A.J. (1982). New Antimicrobials. Br. J. hosp. Med., 27, 136-142.

Garrod, L.P., Lambert, H.P. and O'Grady, F. (1981). Antibiotic and Chemotherapy. Churchill Livingstone, Edinburgh and London.

Selwyn, S.(1976). Rational Choice of Penicillins and Cephalosporins Based on Parallel In-vitro and In-vivo Tests. Lancet, 2, 616-619.

Selwyn, S. (1979a). Pioneer Work on the 'Penicillin Phenomenon', 1870-1876. J. antimicrob. Chemother., 5,249-255.

Selwyn, S. (1979b). The Development of a Hospital Antibiotic Policy in England. In Antibiotics and Hospitals.(eds. C. Grassi and G. Ostini). Alan R. Liss, New York.

Selwyn, S. (1980a). Mechanisms and Range of Activity of Penicillins and Cephalosporins. In The Beta-lactam Antibiotics: Penicillins and Cephalosporins in Perspective. Hodder and Stoughton, London.

Selwyn, S. (1980b). Discovery and Evolution of Penicillins and Cephalosporins. In The Beta-lactam Antibiotics: Penicillins and Cephalosporins in Perspective. Hodder and Stoughton, London.

Selwyn, S. (1980c). Clinical Compendium of Penicillins and Cephalosporins. In The Beta-lactam Antibiotics: Penicillins and Cephalosporins in Perspective. Hodder and Stoughton, London.

Selwyn, S. (1980d). Beta-lactamases in Practice. In The Beta-lactam Antibiotics: Penicillins and Cephalosporins in Perspective. Hodder and Stoughton, London.

Selwyn, S. (1980e). The Role of Beta-lactam Agents in Antibiotic Policies and Strategy. In The Beta-lactam Antibiotics: Penicillins and Cephalosporins in Perspective. Hodder and Stoughton, London.

Selwyn, S. (1981). The Topical Treatment of Skin Infections. In Skin Microbiology: Relevance to Clinical Infection. (eds. H.I. Maibach and R. Aly). Springer-Verlag. New York.

Selwyn, S. (1982). The Evolution of Broad Spectrum Penicillins. J. antimicrob. Chemother., 9, Suppl. B., 1-10.

Slocombe, B., Basker, M.J., Bentley, P.H., Clayton, J.P., Cole, M. Comber, K.R., Dixon, R.A., Edmondson, R.A., Jackson, D., Merrikin, D.J. and Sutherland, R. (1981). BRL 17421, a Novel β-lactam Antibiotic, Highly Resistant to β-lactamases, Giving High and Prolonged Serum Levels in Humans. Antimicrob. Agents Chemother., 20, 38-46.

Sykes, R.B. and Phillips, I. (1981). Azthreonam, a Synthetic Monobactam. J. antimicrob. Chemother., 8, Suppl. E.

Symposium (1977). Fosfomycin: Laboratory Studies. Chemother. 23, Suppl. 1.

Antibiotics as probes of ribosomal structure and function

E Cundliffe

Department of Biochemistry, University of Leicester
Adrian Building, University Road
Leicester, LE1 7RH, UK

INTRODUCTION

A Working Hypothesis

Many antibiotics selectively inhibit protein synthesis and, of these, the majority do so by binding directly to ribosomes. In principle, therefore, it ought to be possible to use antibiotics in order to arrive at structure-function relationships within the ribosomes. The working hypothesis underlying this approach is that ribosomal components involved in binding a given drug might also be involved in the process(es) inhibited by that drug. One purpose of this article is to discuss the extent to which this working hypothesis can be justified and to review various ways in which studies involving antibiotics have contributed to our understanding of ribosomal structure and function.

Complexity and Co-operativity within Ribosomes

Ribosomes from E.coli contain over 50 different proteins (with one exception their molecular weights fall within the range 5,000 - 30,000) and 3 species of RNA; the total particle mass being 2.3 megadaltons. Evidently, within such an organelle, there is no shortage of potential sites to which antibiotics might bind and, in attempting to determine their modes of action, the complexity of ribosomal structure poses various problems. For example, many (perhaps all) of the functions of the ribosome are likely to result from co-operative interactions among the proteins and, possibly also, RNA. Thus, some antibiotics might bind to ribosomal components which play relatively minor roles so that resultant inhibitory effects may be incomplete, especially when the partial reactions of protein synthesis are examined in vitro. This could make it difficult unambiguously to determine their modes of action even though those antibiotics might be effective inhibitors of cell growth. Conversely, some ribosomal components might participate in more than one function so that antibiotics which bind to them might exert multiple effects. Finally, it is even possible that some proteins play no active role whatever in mature ribosomes. Their function might be to direct assembly of the particle or to aid in the processing of ribosomal RNA. Antibiotics which bind to such proteins might not inhibit protein synthesis at all but might, instead, block the biosynthesis of ribosomes.

Criteria for Choosing Suitable Inhibitors

In choosing antibiotics for inclusion in these studies, those whose modes of action are securely established should be preferred even though other compounds might be more important in the clinical context. For a review of antibiotic action against ribosomes, see Cundliffe (1981). Ideally also, suitable drugs should bind to ribosomes firmly and with 1:1 stoichiometry thereby facilitating binding studies while, at the same time, reducing the likelihood that they might exert multiple effects. This stipulation eliminates a great many antibiotics which bind rather loosely to ribosomes and are readily washed away when the latter are subjected to centrifugation, filtration or column chromatography. To circumvent such problems, some drugs have been derivatized to produce affinity analogues able to react covalently with ribosomal components. Doubtless, such analogues (in particular, photoactivatable ones) will feature prominently in the characterization of antibiotic-target sites in ribosomes. However, to date, their use has been complicated by various methodological problems - most notably that of establishing the significance of the labelling patterns observed. For a review, see Cooperman (1980).

THIOSTREPTON : A MODEL ANTIBIOTIC

For the various reasons outlined above, the choice of suitable inhibitors in this context is rather limited. However one compound, the peptide antibiotic thiostrepton, satisfies most of the crucial criteria and has been studied in some detail. This drug is atypical in that it binds very tightly to ribosomes i.e. at least three orders of magnitude more tightly than does, for example, chloramphenicol. Moreover, the mode of action of thiostrepton is known in detail. Crucially, it is relatively easy to re-assemble in vitro, from separated components, ribosomes capable of supporting the reaction upon which assays of the action of thiostrepton are based. That reaction involves hydrolysis of GTP catalysed jointly by the ribosome and the protein elongation factor G (factor EFG). Normally, this process is coupled to polypeptide synthesis so that one molecule of GTP is cleaved (during the so-called "transloca-tion" reaction) following incorporation of each aminoacid residue into peptide linkage. However, in vitro in the absence of mRNA, tRNA or other components required for protein synthesis, ribosomes and factor EFG catalyse "uncoupled" cleavage of GTP. Neither the ribosome nor the factor can, alone, support such hydrolysis nor is it clear which of the two constitutes the GTPase per se and which the activator. Nevertheless, this reaction is powerfully inhibited by thiostrepton and affords a convenient assay for its action. Other ribosomal reactions, each involving the binding of a protein factor, are also sensitive to thiostrepton. The precise relation-ship between the sites at which these reactions occur is not known but it is feasible that thiostrepton blockades a ribosomal domain utilised in common by such protein factors. For a review, see Cundliffe (1981).

Binding of Thiostrepton to Ribosomes

Thiostrepton binds with 1:1 stoichiometry to bacterial ribo-somes or their 50S subunits. Binding is non-covalent (the drug can be removed from ribosomes by extraction with organic solvents) but is remarkably tight and no precise value for the dissociation constant has been determined. The first evidence that protein L11 is somehow involved in the thiostrepton-binding site came when protein-deficient "core" particles, prepared by exposure of ribo-somal 50S subunits to 4M LiCl, were found to bind the drug if supplemented with protein L11 (Highland et al., 1975). These data should now be re-interpreted to show that high affinity binding is dependent upon the presence of protein L11; thiostrepton undoubt-edly binds to ribosomal core particles but not strongly enough to withstand column chromatography. Studies involving equilibrium dialysis and the use of radiolabelled drug have revealed that thiostrepton does not bind to protein L11 (M. Stark and E. Cund-liffe, unpublished data). Rather, the primary binding site is on 23S ribosomal RNA to which thiostrepton binds more tightly than does chloramphenicol to intact ribosomes. However, in the addi-tional presence of protein L11, the binding affinity is greatly enhanced and approaches that observed with intact ribosomes (Thompson et al., 1979). When complexes of E.coli 23S RNA with protein L11 were incubated with ribonuclease, an oligonucleotide 61 residues long was protected from digestion (Schmidt et al., 1981). This RNA fragment rebound specifically to protein L11 and thiostrepton bound to the resultant complex (Table 1). The

Table 1.   Thiostrepton binds to the complex of
            23S RNA with protein L11, even after
            digestion with T_1 ribonuclease.

Order of additions	Binding ratio[a]
23S RNA alone	0.08
23S RNA plus L11	0.95
23S RNA plus T_1 then L11	0.18
23S RNA plus L11 then T_1	0.81

[a] pmol ^{35}S-thiostrepton bound/pmol RNA

nucleotide sequence of the protected RNA fragment, which evidently
contains the attachment site for thiostrepton, is given in Figure
1. In intact 23S RNA from E.coli, this oligonucleotide is located
about one-third of the way in from the 5'-terminus. The secondary
structure given in Figure 1 is compatible with other models (Glotz
et al., 1981; Branlant et al., 1981; Noller et al., 1981). As
discussed below, methylation of residue adenosine-1067 within this
oligonucleotide abolishes the binding of thiostrepton to ribosomes.
This presumably locates the binding site for thiostrepton within
the larger stem-and-loop structure illustrated in Figure 1.

Ribosomes of Thiostrepton-resistant Mutants

Direct binding studies, as discussed above, can be comple-
mented by the examination of antibiotic-resistant mutants,
particularly those containing altered ribosomes. Such mutants,
arising spontaneously and selected for resistance to thiostrepton,
have been obtained from Bacillus megaterium (Cundliffe et al.,
1979) and from Bacillus subtilis (Wienen et al., 1979). These
organisms were employed since thiostrepton does not normally penetrate into Gram-negative organisms such as E.coli. However,
ribosomes from the latter are fully sensitive to the drug in vitro
and were used in the binding studies described above.

Thiostrepton-resistant mutants are not totally insensitive
to the drug; indeed, laboratory mutants selected on any drug do
not commonly display total resistance. Nevertheless, they are
markedly less sensitive than wild-type and similar comments apply

Figure 1. Nucleotide sequence of a fragment of E.coli 23S ribosomal RNA, protected by protein L11 from ribonuclease digestion.

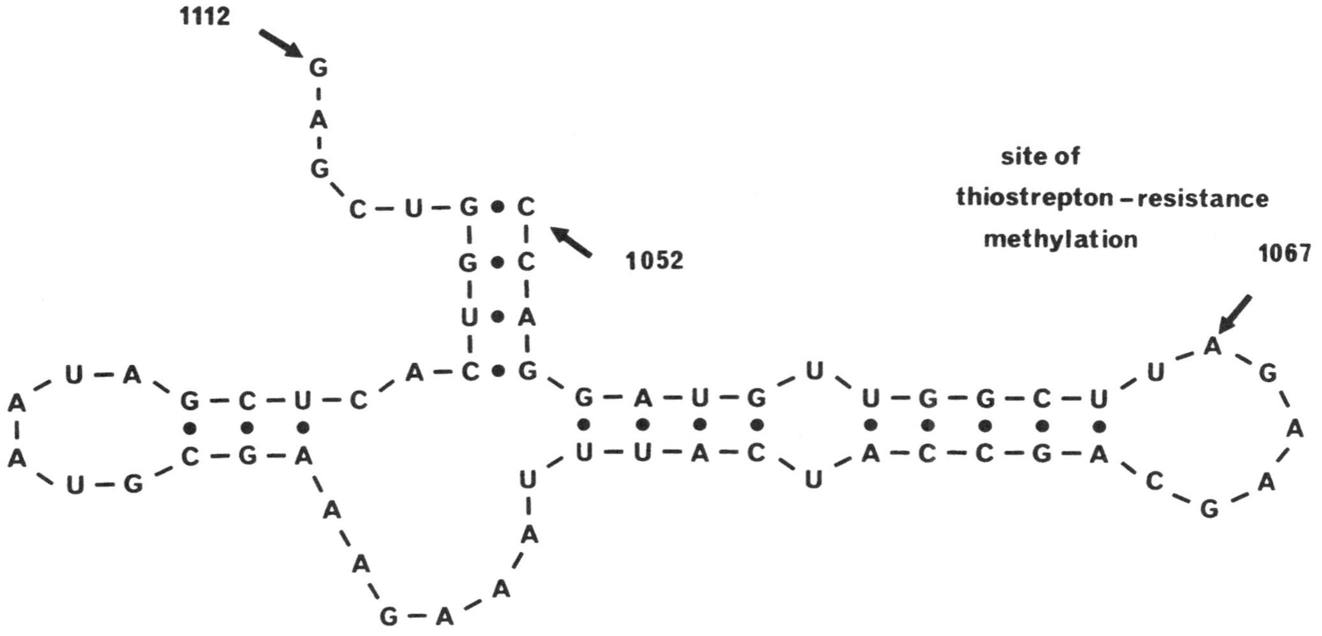

site of
thiostrepton-resistance
methylation

1067

1052

1112

to the properties of their ribosomes when assayed in vitro. When
the ribosomal proteins from such strains were subjected to two-
dimensional electrophoresis in polyacrylamide gels and compared
with those from wild-type, they appeared to lack a single protein
from the 50S subunit. This was confirmed by rigorous immunological examination and the missing protein was shown to be
homologous with E.coli protein L11 (Cundliffe et al., 1979;
Wienen et al., 1979). Fortuitously, when the protein in question
(designated BM-L11) was purified from B.megaterium wild-type, it
proved possible in vitro to re-insert it directly into ribosomes
from thiostrepton-resistant mutants. The reconstituted ribosomes
behaved as wild-type hence, this technique (amounting to in vitro
complementation) could be exploited to determine the biological
role(s) of protein (BM)L11.

Functions of Ribosomal Protein (BM)L11

Thiostrepton-resistant mutants of B.megaterium grow much more
slowly than wild-type and this characteristic is reflected in the
relative efficiencies with which the ribosomes from different
strains support protein synthesis in vitro. However, following
reconstitution with protein BM-L11, ribosomes from a thiostrepton-
resistant strain were indistinguishable from those of wild-type
both in synthetic activity and in response to thiostrepton
(Cundliffe et al., 1979). Examination of the partial reactions
of protein synthesis revealed that ribosomes from the mutant were
specifically defective in their ability to catalyse the uncoupled
hydrolysis of GTP in association with factor EF G (Stark and
Cundliffe, 1979a). Otherwise, they appeared to be fully active
in their capacity to promote peptide bond formation, to bind
aminoacyl-tRNA from the ternary complex with factor EF Tu and GTP
and to hydrolyse GTP during binding of aminoacyl-tRNA. The ability
of the ribosomal subunits to associate was not notably affected
nor was the binding of guanine nucleotides in the presence of
factor EF G. This suggested a role for protein BM-L11 in GTP
hydrolysis (as opposed to GTP binding) catalysed by the ribosome
and factor EF G. Significantly, when ribosomes from the mutant
were supplemented with purified protein BM-L11 they were restored
to full GTPase activity; this process also became fully sensitive
to thiostrepton (Figure 2).

Thiostrepton-resistant mutants also exhibit relaxed control
of RNA synthesis. That is, they do not reduce their rate of RNA
synthesis under conditions of aminoacid starvation. Normally,
under such circumstances, guanosine penta- and tetra-phosphates
are produced (by pyrophosphate transfer from ATP onto the 3'-
hydroxyl group of GTP or GDP) in a ribosome-dependent reaction

Figure 2.　Role of ribosomal protein BM-L11 in factor-dependent
GTP hydrolysis.

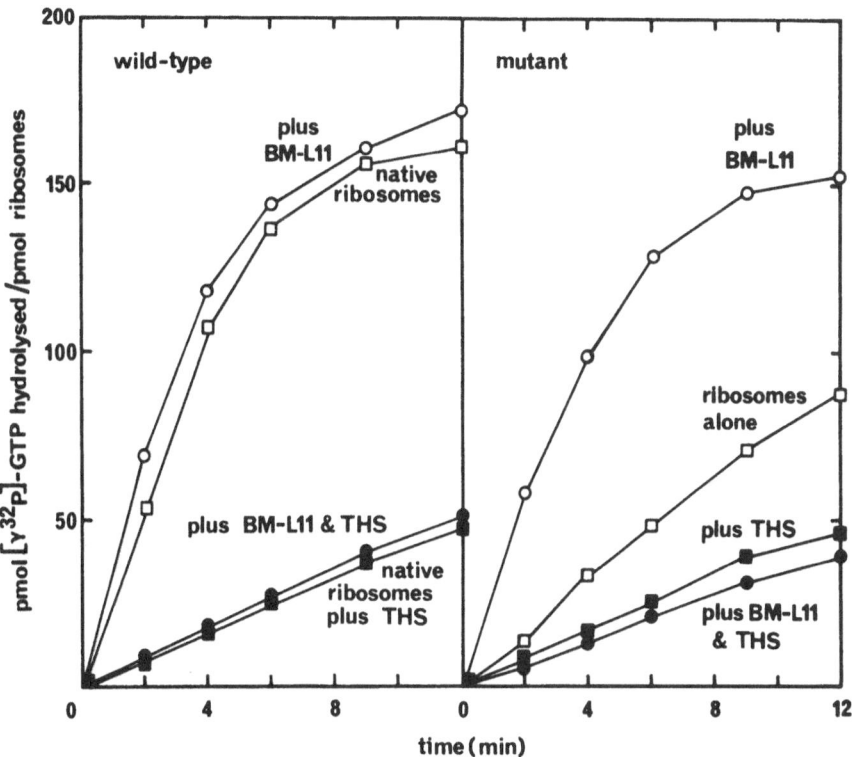

Ribosomes from B.megaterium wild-type or from a thiostrepton-
resistant strain lacking ribosomal protein BM-L11 were incubated
with factor EF G from E.coli in the presence of GTP. Some
batches of ribosomes were previously incubated with a 4-fold
molar excess of protein BM-L11. Thiostrepton, when present, was
used at approximately 12-fold molar excess over ribosomes. Data
taken from Stark and Cundliffe, (1979a). THS = thiostrepton.

involving stringent factor (a non-ribosomal protein) and mRNA-cognate deacylated tRNA. The resultant guanosine polyphosphates are regulatory nucleotides which modify the activity of RNA polymerase - the so-called "stringent" response. Thiostrepton-resistant mutants of B.subtilis did not produce guanosine poly-phosphates in vivo in response to aminoacid starvation nor could their ribosomes support such synthesis in cell-free systems (Smith et al., 1978). However, thiostrepton-sensitive revertants had regained the stringent response and their ribosomes possessed the previously-missing protein. Cause and effect were established when ribosomes from thiostrepton-resistant mutants of B.megaterium were supplemented with protein BM-L11 in vitro. This restored their ability to support guanosine polyphosphate production (Stark and Cundliffe, 1979b) and suggested an indispensable role for protein BM-L11, either in the binding or action of stringent fac-tor.

The homology between proteins BM-L11 from B.megaterium and L11 from E.coli also extends to function. Thus, all the effects described above,resulting from the re-addition of protein BM-L11 to ribosomes from thiostrepton-resistant mutants, were also pro-duced by supplementation with protein L11 (Stark et al., 1980). Evidently, proteins L11 and BM-L11 are both physically and func-tionally homologous.

Localization of a Functional Ribosomal Site

The results presented above establish an intimate relation-ship between the site of action of thiostrepton and the ribosomal neighbourhood containing protein L11. Localization of this functional site on the ribosomal surface has been achieved by immuno electron microscopy using antibodies raised against protein L11 and against thiostrepton. Ribosomal 50S subunits were decora-ted with antibody or, alternatively, subunit-dimers held together by bivalent antibody were recovered from sucrose density-gradients. In either case, electron microscopy revealed that antibody had attached to the ribosomal 50S subunit at a central position on the concave surface which forms an interface with the 30S subunit in the intact ribosome (Figure 3; see also Stöffler et al., 1980). The proximity of these sites to the ribosomal "stalk" is signifi-cant since the latter contains the tetrameric protein L7/L12 which has been cross-linked to protein L11 in situ (Expert-Bezançon et al., 1976). Protein L7/L12 is apparently required for the inter-action of proteins, such as factors EF G and EF Tu, with the ribosome and is therefore a component of the functional domain which also contains protein L11 and which is perturbed by thio-strepton.

72

Figure 3.   The ribosomal binding site for thiostrepton.

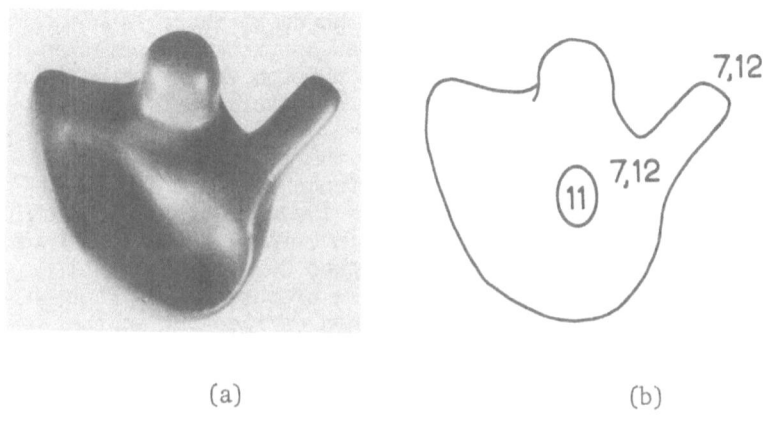

(a)   (b)

(a)   The 50S ribosomal subunit according to Lake (1976).
       Model kindly provided by Jim Lake.

(b)   Schematic representation of the 50S ribosomal subunit to
       show the location of proteins L7/L12 (Strycharz et al.,
       1978) and of protein L11 (Stöffler et al., 1980). The oval
       represents the approximate site of attachment of anti-
       thiostrepton antibody (Stöffler et al., 1980).

THE WORKING HYPOTHESIS REVIEWED

Thiostrepton inhibits various reactions dependent upon the
binding of protein factors to the ribosome. Two such reactions
(namely, GTP hydrolysis promoted by factor EF G and guanosine
polyphosphate production dependent on stringent factor) have been
studied here and three salient points can be made in surveying
the results. Firstly, thiostrepton binds to a single ribosomal
site; secondly, protein L11 plays an important role in both the
reactions inhibited by thiostrepton and thirdly, thiostrepton
binds to 23S rRNA within the binding site for protein L11. Since
ribosomes contain only a single copy of protein L11, it is proposed that thiostrepton interferes with protein synthesis by dis-
torting or abolishing functions of that protein. In other words,
thiostrepton acts where it binds with no evident propagation of
its effects to distant sites on the ribosome. Presumably, since

thiostrepton does not displace protein L11 from the ribosome, there must be some change in the conformation of that protein in situ since its functions are attenuated. Also, it is possible that the secondary and/or tertiary structure of 23S RNA is distorted when thiostrepton binds to it. However, there is no necessity to postulate that the drug causes gross conformational changes of the type which might spread through the ribosome like shock waves and give rise to multiple, allosteric effects.

This line of reasoning emphasises the relative rigidity of the ribosome without denying the occurrence of local structural re-arrangements. It therefore supports the concept of ribosomal neighbourhoods, constituting discrete functional domains, any or all of which might be selectively attacked by different antibiotics. Studies of the modes of action of antibiotics (not only upon protein synthesis) have usually been carried out in the belief that such drugs would ultimately be found to possess single "primary" modes of action. In the case of antibiotics acting upon ribosomes, such studies are now seen to be based upon more than an article of faith.

AUTOIMMUNITY IN THE THIOSTREPTON-PRODUCER

Thiostrepton is produced by Streptomyces azureus, a Gram-positive bacterium. Although streptomycetes in general are extremely sensitive to the action of thiostrepton, S.azureus is totally resistant to the drug as are its ribosomes when assayed in cell-free protein synthesis. Ribosomes from S.azureus do not bind thiostrepton at all although they do contain a protein, immunologically related to E.coli protein L11 (G. Stöffler, personal communication), which together with 23S RNA from E.coli can constitute a high affinity binding site for the drug. Eventually, it was established that S.azureus possesses a methylase enzyme which acts upon 23S rRNA and renders ribosomes selectively resistant to thiostrepton (Cundliffe, 1978). The "thiostrepton-resistance methylase" acts upon free rRNA but not upon 50S ribosomal subunits (Thompson and Cundliffe, 1981) and a typical example of its effects is given in Table 2. This enzyme is produced constitutively by S.azureus and presumably acts upon rRNA at an early stage during or after transcription. A single residue of 2'-O-methyladenosine is produced (Cundliffe and Thompson, 1979) and, with E.coli 23S RNA as substrate, this is located at position 1067 in the polynucleotide chain (J. Thompson, F. Schmidt and E. Cundliffe, unpublished data). This lies within the RNA fragment protected by protein L11 (Figure 1) and, presumably, indicates precisely where thiostrepton binds.

Table 2.   Properties of reconstituted 50S ribosomal sub-
           units containing 23S RNA subjected to the action
           of the thiostrepton-resistance methylase.

50S particles	Thiostrepton[a] input	GTP hydrolysis[b]
Native	0	135
	3	6
Reconstituted with	0	170
unmethylated RNA	3	24
Reconstituted with	0	185
methylated RNA	30	175

[a]molar excess over 50S particles

[b]pmol ^{32}P-GTP hydrolysed/min/pmol 50S particles

Total ribosomal RNA from E.coli was treated with the
thiostrepton-resistance methylase in the presence and
absence of S-adenosyl-methionine. The RNA was then
supplemented with total 50S subunit proteins and the
reconstituted particles assayed for their ability to
hydrolyse GTP in the presence of factor EF G. Native
50S subunits were used as controls. All were assayed
in the presence of a 4-fold excess of 30S subunits
which, alone, were without activity.

A conceptually similar enzyme is responsible for resistance
to erythromycin in the producer, Streptomyces erythreus (Skinner
and Cundliffe, 1982). In this case, dimethylation of 23S RNA
with the production of a single residue of N^6,N^6-dimethyladenine
determines resistance. As yet, the site of action of the "erythromycin-resistance methylase" is not known. No other examples
of ribosomal modification as a means of self defence are known.
Hence, it remains to be seen how widespread this stratagem is and
how varied the mechanisms are. Obviously, enzymes such as the
thiostrepton- and erythromycin-resistance methylases are valuable
biochemical tools. By pinpointing antibiotic-binding sites, they
should greatly aid the localization and characterization of functional domains within the ribosome.

ACKNOWLEDGEMENT

Work in the author's laboratory is supported by the Medical Research Council.

REFERENCES

Branlant, C., Krol, A., Machatt, M.A., Pouyet, J., Ebel, J-P., Edwards, K. and Kössel, H. (1981). Primary and Secondary Structures of Escherichia coli MRE 600 23S Ribosomal RNA. Comparison with Models of Secondary Structure for Maize Chloroplast 23S rRNA and for Large Portions of Mouse and Human 16S Mitochondrial rRNAs. Nuc. Acids Res., 9, 4303-4324.

Cooperman, B.S. (1980). Functional Sites on the E.coli Ribosome as Defined by Affinity Labelling. In Ribosomes : Structure, Function and Genetics (eds. G. Chambliss, G.R. Craven, J. Davies, K. Davis, L. Kahan and M. Nomura). University Park Press, Baltimore.

Cundliffe, E. (1978). Mechanism of Resistance to Thiostrepton in the Producing-Organism Streptomyces azureus. Nature, 272, 792-795.

Cundliffe, E. (1981). Antibiotic Inhibitors of Ribosome Function. In The Molecular Basis of Antibiotic Action. E.F. Gale, E. Cundliffe, P.E. Reynolds, M.H. Richmond and M.J. Waring. Wiley, Chichester.

Cundliffe, E., Dixon, P., Stark, M., Stöffler, G., Ehrlich, R., Stöffler-Meilicke, R. and Cannon, M. (1979). Ribosomes in Thiostrepton-Resistant Mutants of Bacillus megaterium Lacking a Single 50S Subunit Protein. J.Mol.Biol., 132, 235-252.

Cundliffe, E. and Thompson, J. (1979). Ribose Methylation and Resistance to Thiostrepton. Nature, 278, 859-861.

Expert-Bezançon, A., Barritault, D., Milet, M. and Hayes, D.H. (1976). Close Proximity of Escherichia coli 50S Subunit Proteins L7/L12 and L10 and L11. J.Mol.Biol.,108, 781-787.

Glotz, C., Zwieb, C., Brimacombe, R., Edwards, K. and Kössel, H. (1981). Secondary Structure of the Large Ribosomal RNA from Escherichia coli, Zea mays Chloroplast, and Human and Mouse Mitochondrial Ribosomes. Nuc. Acids Res., 9, 3287-3306.

Highland, J.H., Howard, G.A., Ochsner, E., Stöffler, G., Hasenbank, R. and Gordon, J. (1975). Identification of a Ribosomal Protein Necessary for Thiostrepton Binding to E.coli Ribosomes. J. Biol. Chem., 250, 1141-1145.

Lake, J.A. (1976). Ribosomal Structure Determined by Electron Microscopy of Escherichia coli Small Subunits, Large Subunits and Monomeric Ribosomes. J. Mol. Biol., 105, 131-159.

Noller, H.J., Kop, J., Wheaton, V., Brosius, J., Gutell, R.R., Kopylov, A.M., Dohme, F., Herr, W., Stahl, D.A., Gupta, R. and Woese, C.R. (1981) Secondary Structure Model for 23S Ribosomal RNA. Nuc. Acids Res., 9, 6167-6189.

Skinner, R.H. and Cundliffe, E. (1982). Dimethylation of Adenine and the Resistance of Streptomyces erythreus to Erythromycin. J. Gen. Microbiol., in press.

Smith, I., Paress, P. and Pestka, S. (1978). Thiostrepton-Resistant Mutants Exhibit Relaxed Synthesis of RNA. Proc. Nat. Acad. Sci., USA, 75, 5993-5997.

Stark, M.J.R. and Cundliffe, E. (1979a). On the Biological Role of Ribosomal Protein BM-L11 of B. megaterium, Homologous with E.coli Ribosomal Protein L11. J. Mol. Biol., 134, 767-779.

Stark, M.J.R. and Cundliffe, E. (1979b). Requirement for Ribosomal Protein BM-L11 in Stringent Control of RNA Synthesis in Bacillus megaterium. Eur. J. Biochem., 102, 101-105.

Stark, M.J.R., Cundliffe, E., Dijk, J. and Stöffler, G. (1980). Functional Homology Between E. coli Ribosomal Protein L11 and B. megaterium Protein BM-L11. Molec. Gen. Genet., 180, 11-15.

Stöffler, G., Bald, R., Kastner, B., Lührmann, R., Stöffler-Meilicke, M. and Tischendorf, G. (1980). Structural Organization of the Escherichia coli Ribosome and Localization of Functional Domains. In Ribosomes : Structure, Function and Genetics. (eds. G. Chambliss, G.R. Craven, J. Davies, K. Davis, L. Kahan and M. Nomura). University Park Press, Baltimore.

Strycharz, W.A., Nomura, M. and Lake, J.A. (1978). Ribosomal Proteins L7/L12 Localized at a Single Region of the Large Subunit by Immune Electron Microscopy. J. Mol. Biol., 126, 123-140.

Thompson, J. and Cundliffe, E. (1981). Purification and Properties of an RNA Methylase Produced by Streptomyces azureus and Involved in Resistance to Thiostrepton. J. Gen. Microbiol., 124, 291-297.

Thompson, J., Cundliffe, E. and Stark, M. (1979). Binding of Thiostrepton to a Complex of 23S rRNA with Ribosomal Protein L11. Eur. J. Biochem., 98, 261-265.

Wienen, B., Ehrlich, R., Stöffler-Meilicke, M., Stöffler, G., Smith, I., Weiss, D., Vince, R. and Pestka, S. (1979). Ribosomal Protein Alterations in Thiostrepton- and Micrococcin-Resistant Mutants of Bacillus subtilis. J. Biol. Chem., 254, 8031-8041.

Mechanisms of drug resistance

Professor J T Smith

The Microbiology Section, Department of Pharmaceutics
The School of Pharmacy, University of London
Brunswick Square, London WC1N 1AX, UK

Resistance to antibiotics in bacteria has shown an explosive increase in recent years, which in some instances has more than kept pace with the commercial production and clinical use of antibiotics and chemotherapeutic agents.

Although it is known that bacteria can mutate to become drug-resistant this process is generally not responsible for the resistance of clinical bacterial isolates to antibiotics. One reason for this is perhaps because such mutants often exhibit reduced pathogenicity (Knox and Smith, 1961). On the other hand, clinical antibiotic resistance is usually caused by the presence of antibiotic resistance plasmids, and hence by definition the presence of such R-plasmids must have little or no deleterious effect on pathogenicity.

R-plasmids usually confer drug resistance by causing their bacterial hosts to inactivate antibiotics. Sometimes the resistance mechanism is that of impermeability and in the remaining cases the mechanism is the insusceptible target site variety. This contrasts with the situation found in laboratory-selected chromosomal mutants where the insusceptible target site mechanism is the most common, followed by impermeability while drug inactivation never arises. Thus such mutants are of little use where the study of clinical antibiotic resistance is concerned.

The fact that the de novo appearance of an antibiotic inactivating enzyme by mutation has not been reported is not surprising because mutations fall into two classes; base changes and nucleotide deletions. The former alter only one amino acid in one protein while the latter delete a small section of amino acids from a protein. Hence neither of these mutational mechanisms could add a completely new protein to a mutant. For example, an enzyme of

79

molecular weight of about 30,000 Daltons would be comprised of 250 amino acids and therefore 750 nucleotides would require to be added to the genetic complement of the cell by mutation. Clearly this could not occur. On the other hand, if an organism already produces low levels of an enzyme, then mutation can alter the control of its synthesis so that mutants can arise producing so much enzyme that significant antibiotic resistance now occurs. This indeed is the case with Shigella sonnei where its chromosomal β-lactamase production is normally not sufficient to cause significant β lactam antibiotic resistance. However, mutants do arise clinically that produce 80 to 180 times more chromosomal β lactamase to cause the failure of therapy with susceptible β-lactam antibiotics. (Smith, et al, 1974).

Such examples are rare and generally speaking the resistance mechanisms of R-plasmids in clinical isolates differ greatly from the mechanisms of resistance found in laboratory-selected chromosomal mutants. This stems from the fact that bacteria which harbour R-plasmids are partial diploids in that they possess not only genes specifying resistance on the plasmid but also another set of genes on the chromosome specifying sensitivity to the same drug. This contrasts with the situation in chromosomal mutants where the sensitivity genes on the chromosome have been completely altered by the effects of the mutation to become resistance genes and hence the organism has been changed from a pure sensitive genotype to a pure resistant genotype. Although with such mutants the insusceptible target site mechanism of resistance is very efficient, this mechanism could not operate if mediated by an R-plasmid, at least where resistance to drugs inhibiting ribosomal function are concerned. The reason for this is that during protein synthesis many ribosomes are simultaneously translated into protein on each strand of messenger RNA, i.e. as polysomes. Hence any resistant ribosomes (coded for by a hypothetical plasmid) would be prevented from functioning by their association with drug-affected sensitive ribosomes (coded by the chromosome) on the same strand of messenger RNA. Nevertheless, R-plasmids found in Staphylococci and Streptococci have overcome this drawback to cause macrolide and lincosaminide resistance by conferring on their hosts the synthesis of a methylating enzyme which dimethylates one or two adenine residues of the 23S ribosomal RNA of the 50S ribosome subunit (Lai et al, 1973; Courvalin et al, 1972). Such adenine methylation occurs to every ribosome in the cell and since methylated ribosomes no longer can bind the drugs the bacteria are hence rendered resistant.

It is also hard to imagine how a plasmid could confer resistance to drugs acting on cell wall synthesis should it convey the insusceptible target site mechanism of resistance. If such a situation was to occur then the plasmid would be unlikely to confer resistance because even if only a small proportion of mucopeptide was synthesized under the influence of an antibiotic-sensitive mucopeptide transpeptidase mediated by the chromosome then the antibiotics could inhibit the sensitive transpeptidase so causing the formation of weakened areas of mucopeptide through which escape of cell contents could occur to cause cell death.

In a similar vein it is doubtful whether plasmids could confer antibiotic resistance via a straightforward impermeability mechanism. In this situation the cell membrane could be a mosaic of impermeable membrane (mediated by the plasmid) and permeable membrane (mediated by the chromosome) through which the drug could still gain access to the cell. R-plasmids in Gram negative bacteria and in Staphylococci do confer impermeability to tetracyclines but the mechanism is by no means straightforward. The plasmid in these bacteria operates by causing its host to synthesize one or more special proteins which migrate to all the cell membrane tetracycline uptake sites and so block the ingress of the drug (Levy and McMurry, 1974; Chopra and Howe, 1978). This mechanism, in common with that described earlier for macrolide resistance in Gram positive cocci, hence circumvents the problem of cells harbouring R-plasmids being partial diploids with respect to the genes for antibiotic sensitivity and resistance.

The mechanisms of resistance of bacteria harbouring R-plasmids vary in relation to each individual group of antibiotics. With R-plasmid mediated resistance to the β-lactam antibiotics we found that when the enzymological properties of the β-lactamases mediated by such R-plasmids were analyzed an enzymic type termed TEM predominated, and we concluded that "the ubiquity of the structural gene for the TEM-like enzyme demonstrates its evolutionary success which probably results from its ability to be translocated from one replicon to another." (Hedges et al, 1974.) Later the term transposon was proposed for such mobile R-plasmid antibiotic resistance genes (Hedges and Jacob, 1974). Subsequently the DNA segment containing the TEM β-lactamase gene (termed transposon A, but now called Tn1) was shown to be bounded by inverted repeated DNA sequences that possibly facilitate the exchange of this particular DNA molecule between R-plasmids (Heffron et al, 1975). Other antibiotic resistance genes of R-plasmids (such as tetracycline, chloramphenicol and kanamycin) have since been classified as transposons (Cohen, 1976).

81

The first report of an altered target site mechanism of R-plasmid mediated resistance to any chemotherapeutic agent in Gram-negative bacteria was when we described the trimethoprim-resistant dihydrofolate reductase of R388 (Amyes and Smith, 1974). Since then other types of trimethoprim-resistant dihydrofolate reductases have appeared. One of these enzymic types is appearing at high frequency in both animal and human trimethoprim-resistant bacteria (Broad and Smith, 1982). It would hence seem that another trans-poson is at work disseminating trimethoprim resistance not only between plasmids but also from animals to humans.

The mechanisms of resistance mediated by R-plasmids to amino-glycoside antibiotics are almost exclusively enzymic inactivation; either by acetylation, phosphorylation or adenylylation. There are many of these enzymes; each having its own substrate specif-icity, and hence resistance spectrum, among the aminoglycoside antibiotics. However, when bacteria harbouring R-plasmids are grown in media containing aminoglycoside antibiotics to which their plasmids confer resistance it is found that little or no significant diminution of the concentration of the drug in the medium can be detected. This situation contrasts with plasmid-mediated penicillin or chloramphenicol resistance where all the antibiotic in the medium is destroyed by the plasmid-mediated drug inactivating enzymes prior to bacterial multiplication (Reynolds and Smith, 1979). Therefore it would seem that the resistance mechanism mediated by the plasmids to aminoglycoside antibiotics cannot be solely ascribed to inactivation. However, as there is no doubt that drug modification by these enzymes does cause resistance it would seem that the actual mechanism of resistance could be due to the trace amounts of modified drug being able to block the uptake of active drug through the outer layers of the bacteria harbouring such plasmids. Thus resistance to amino-glycoside antibiotics may be a consequence of plasmid-mediated drug inactivation which leads ultimately to cellular impermeability.

References

Amyes, S.G.B. and Smith, J.T. (1974). R-factor trimethoprim resistance mechanism: an insusceptible target site. Biochemical and Biophysical Research Communications, 58, 412-418.

Broad, D.F. and Smith, J.T. (1982). Classification of trimethoprim-resistant dihydrofolate reductase mediated by R-plasmids by iso-electric focussing. European Journal of Biochemistry. Accepted for publication.

Chopra, I. and Howe, T.G.B. (1978). Bacterial resistance to the tetracyclines. Microbiological Reviews, 42, 707-724.

Cohen, S.N. (1976). Transposable genetic elements and plasmid evolution. Nature, 263, 731-738.

Courvalin, P.M., Carlier, C. and Chabbert, Y.A. (1972). Plasmid-linked tetracycline and erythromycin resistance in group D "Streptococcus". Annals of the Institut Pasteur, 123, 755-759.

Hedges, R.W., Datta, N., Kontomichalou, P. and Smith, J.T. (1974). Molecular specificities of R-factor determined beta lactamases: correlation with plasmid compatibility. Journal of Bacteriology, 117, 56-62.

Hedges, R.W. and Jacob, A.E. (1974). Transposition of ampicillin resistance from RP4 to other replicons. Molecular and General Genetics, 132, 31-40.

Heffron, F., Rubens, C. and Falkow, S. (1975). Translocation of a plasmid sequence which mediates ampicillin resistance: Molecular nature and specificity of insertion. Proceedings of the National Academy of Sciences U.S.A., 72, 3623-3627.

Knox, R. and Smith, J.T. (1961). The nature of penicillin resistance in Staphylococci. Lancet, ii, 520-522.

Lai, C.J., Dahlberg, J. and Weisblum, B. (1973). Structure of an inducibly methylatable nucleotide sequence in 23 S ribosomal ribonucleic acid from erythromycin-resistant Staphylococcus aureus. Biochemistry, 12, 457-460.

Levy, S.B. and McMurry, L. (1974). Detection of an inducible membrane protein associated with R-factor mediated tetracycline resistance. Biochemical and Biophysical Research Communications, 56, 1060-1068.

Reynolds, A.V. and Smith, J.T. (1979). Enzymes which modify aminoglycoside antibiotics. Recent Advances in Infection, 1, 165-181.

Smith, J.T., Bremner, D.A. and Datta, N. (1974). Ampicillin resistance of Shigella Sonnei. Antimicrobial Agents and Chemotherapy, 6, 418-421.

New strategies in the search for antiprotozoal drugs

Professor B A Newton

Medical Research Council Unit for Biochemical
Parasitology
The Molteno Institute, University of Cambridge
Dowing Street, Cambridge, CB2 3EE, UK

INTRODUCTION

More than one hundred and twenty species of parasitic protozoa (Baker, 1982) are of medical or veterinary importance. In man they have an almost world-wide distribution and, at any one time, probably afflict about a quarter of the worlds population. These parasites may infect the gastrointestinal or urinogenital tracts, central or peripheral nervous systems, muscle or the reticuloendothelial system. Although chemotherapy is inadequate for some of these diseases there are (if we include veterinary compounds) more than forty drugs currently used in their treatment (Klein, 1980), some of them excellent. Clearly it is an impossible task in the space available to review this whole field and to consider strategies in the search for new drugs for such a diverse range of parasites. I have chosen, therefore, to limit my discussion to some new approaches to the chemotherapy of the protozoal diseases included in the UNDP/World Bank/WHO Special Programme for Research and Training in Tropical Diseases which, since it was launched in 1975, has initiated many new research programmes. These diseases include the trypano-somiases (African and S. American), malaria and the leishmaniases.

THE PRESENT SITUATION

In order to appreciate the urgency of the need for new drugs to combat these diseases we must consider, briefly, the present situation. In Africa trypanosomiasis occurs over an area of <u>ca</u>

four million square miles south of the Sahara affecting man and domestic animals and causing wide spread suffering, malnutrition and abandonment of fertile land. It is difficult to obtain accurate estimates of the number of people and animals at risk in more than thirty countries: WHO and FAO have published figures in the range of thirty five to forty million people and upto eighty million cattle. Chemotherapeutic control of trypanosomiasis in man relies on three drugs: suramin, pentamidine and melarsoprol. Ideally treatment should be carried out in hospital because of side effects due to drug toxicity. Treatment of early stage (ie bloodstream infections without CNS involvement) requires four to six weeks, suramin being used for T. rhodesiense and pentamidine for T. gambiense infections. The only drug available for late stage sleeping sickness (ie with CNS involvement) is melarsoprol (Mel B), this drug, introduced in 1946 produces serious side effects (reactive encephalopathy) in 5-10% of cases treated and 2-5% fatalities occur resulting from drug treatment: hospitalization for about a month is essential. The situation is not a lot better for the control of the disease in cattle: four or five drugs are currently used (ethidium, quinapyramine, berenil, pyrithidium and isometamidium) but resistance to all of them has been reported and is often accompanied by cross resistance. No new drugs have been put on the market for about thirty years.

The South American form of trypanosomiasis (Chagas' disease) remains a major health problem, it is most prevalent in Argentina, Brazil, Chile and Venezuela. Thirty five million people live in areas where it is endemic and at least twelve million are believed to be infected. Only two drugs (Nifurtimox and Benznidazole, marketed in 1976 and 1978 respectively) are in use: both produce unpleasant side effects and doubt remains about their effectiveness against chronic cases.

The situation is little better for the leishmaniases: the drug of choice for visceral infections is a pentavalent antimonial - sodium stibogluconate (Pentostam), if an infection does not respond to this treatment an aromatic diamidine such as pentamidine may be used and if this fails the highly toxic fungicide amphotericin B is the last resort. The diffuse cutaneous form of the disease is generally resistant to treatment and constantly relapses. All the antimonials are toxic compounds which have to be administered daily by intravenous injection for ten days and it is not unusual for patients to discontinue therapy because of unpleasant side effects.

The situation with malaria is not quite so gloomy, a number of excellent drugs are available for treatment and prophylaxis, chloroquine and amodiaquine being the cheapest and most effective.

Others include pyrimethamine, primaquine, proguanil and the most recent addition, mefloquin but in spite of the availability of all these drugs the disease still causes more than a million deaths a year and chloroquin resistance in P. falciparum continues to spread. There is a great need for an inexpensive long-acting blood schizontocide which would maintain its effects for at least a month after administration of a single oral dose and for a well-tolerated tissue schizontocide capable of a radical cure of P. vivax and P. ovale infections.

Without exception all the drugs in current use against these diseases have resulted from screening very large numbers of compounds synthesised by the pharmaceutical industry and systematic synthesis of derivatives when a new 'lead substance' has emerged. The fact that few new drugs have come onto the market in the last thirty years reflects the problems of this approach. The success rate is low (ca 1/100,000); many of the lead compounds were identified forty to sixty years ago and variations on these themes have been largely exhausted; systematic synthesis of analogues of active compounds has resulted in chemically related compounds being marketed and the development of drug resistance to one is frequently accompanied by cross resistance to others. Research and development costs continually rise (in 1979 $ US 6–8 million was thought to be a realistic estimate for putting a new drug on the market; development costs for the latest antimalarial (mefloquin) have recently been put at $ US 15 million) and the poverty of the less developed countries makes them an unattractive market (the world market for trypanocidal drugs was recently estimated to be only $ US 12 million p.a.). The result is that only a small and diminishing number of pharmaceutical companies are now actively searching for new drugs to treat these diseases: the number of drug companies with an antimalarial programme is reported to have fallen from fifteen to five in recent years. It is the view of some of us who are concerned with these problems that if, over the last ten to twenty years, fundamental research on the biology of parasites had received funding comparable to screening and chemical synthesis in industry, the new leads that we now so desparately need would have emerged. A number of research funding organizations are now trying to redress the balance a little and in the last decade an increasing number of biochemists, immunologist and geneticists have become involved in the study of host/parasite relationships. Recent work on the structural and metabolic changes which occur during the developmental cycle of parasitic protozoa has brought to light unique features in the cell biology of these organisms which I believe may ultimately provide leads for the development of a new generation of drugs. I will discuss some of these advances and ideas arising from them.

THE SEARCH FOR UNIQUE FEATURES IN THE PHYSIOLOGY OF PARASITIC PROTOZOA

Energy Metabolism

The first indication that there may be unique steps in the
energy metabolism of African trypanosomes came from the classical
comparative study of von Brand and Johnson (1947) in which they
showed that respiration of bloodstream trypomastigotes was
cyanide resistant whereas that of culture forms was not. We know
now that the biogenesis of the mitochondrial respiratory chain is
suppressed in bloodstream forms and that these forms, which are
entirely dependent upon an exogenous supply of carbohydrate,
metabolise glucose by glycolysis involving pathways essentially
similar to those of their hosts with one exception: the NAD^+
reduced in the glyceraldehyde phosphate dehydrogenase step is not
reoxidised by a lactate dehydrogenase, which is missing, but by a
glycerolphosphate shuttle involving two enzymes, an NAD^+ -
dependent glycerol.3.phosphate dehydrogenase and a glycerol.3.
phosphate oxidase (Grant and Sargent, 1960; Opperdoes et al 1977).
The oxidase was initially believed to be essential for energy
production in the absence of a functional mitochondrion and since
it does not occur in mammalian cells it was thought to be an
ideal target for a selective chemotherapeutic agent. Evans and
Brown (1973) showed that m - chlorobenzhydroxamate, a known
inhibitor of oxidases in plants, blocked O_2 uptake by bloodstream
trypanosomes; a number of other aromatic hydroxamic acids (eg
salicylhydroxamic acid, SHAM) were similarly active but when
tested on T. brucei infected rats (Opperdoes et al 1976) at concentrations which gave blood levels of the inhibitor equivalent
to 100 times the K_i for the isolated oxidase no effect on the
parasitaemia was observed. It was subsequently shown that the
failure of SHAM to inhibit parasite growth under these conditions
was due to the existance of an alternative metabolic pathway in
the trypanosomes by which glucose utilization proceeded with net
ATP synthesis and the production of equimolar amounts of pyruvate
and glycerol (Opperdoes et al 1976): it is now thought that this
pathway involves the reversal of the glycerokinase catalyzed
reaction (Opperdoes and Borst, 1977; Hammond and Bowman, 1980).
Clarkson and Brohn (1976) predicted that glycerol should inhibit
this alternative pathway by mass action and showed that a combination of glycerol and SHAM is indeed lethal to T. brucei in
vivo and in vitro: this finding has been confirmed and extended
to other species of African trypanosomes (Fairlamb et al 1977;

Evans et al 1977; Evans and Holland, 1978) but unfortunately the concentration of SHAM/glycerol required to produce a radical cure is very high and very toxic. In an attempt to develop a practical therapeutic regimen glycerol is now being replaced by other polyols and SHAM by other hydroxamates and compounds with iron binding moieties (Clarkson et al 1981) so far without success, but I am sure this approach will be pursued further.

The lesson to be learnt from this investigation is that in seeking new leads for chemotherapy it is not sufficient to identify a unique pathway in a parasite or to find a selective inhibitor for that pathway - one must also establish that the parasite is absolutely dependent upon the pathway and cannot bye-pass it.

In the course of this work on trypanosome energy metabolism it was shown that the enzymes involved in the conversion of glucose to 3.glycerophosphate are located in a microbody-like organelle - named a glycosome (Opperdoes and Borst, 1977), these enzymes are latent and it has been suggested (Opperdoes and Borst, 1977) that the glycosome has evolved to optimize conditions for glycolysis by creating a compartment where high concentrations of substrates are maintained and they suggested that specific translocators may exist to transport certain metabolic intermediates (eg triose phosphate) across the glycosome membrane however, more recent work (Visser and Opperdoes, 1980) casts doubt on this hypothesis. Nevertheless there is evidence for a similar intracellular localization of glycolytic enzymes in T. cruzi and Leishmania (Taylor et al 1980) and since there appears to be no equivalent to the glycosome in mammalian cells it might be considered a potential chemotherapeutic target and further work on this organelle would seem to be justified.

Another aspect of trypanosome and leishmanial metabolism currently attracting attention relates to the inability of these parasites to synthesise haem, as a result they lack the enzyme catalase (Fulton and Spooner, 1956) this has focussed attention on the production and regulation of the intracellular concentration of hydrogen peroxide (H_2O_2), a normal product of aerobic metabolism which is well known to be cytotoxic. Most cells are protected against H_2O_2 by enzymes such as catalase and glutathione (GSH) peroxidase. It has been found that intracellular levels of H_2O_2 in bloodstream forms of T. brucei are about 70 µM (Meshnick et al 1977), a value at least 100-fold higher than that reported in mammalian cells and the therapeutic potential of this situation has been recognised: the parasites should be susceptible to agents which increase intracellular H_2O_2, produce superoxide (O_2^-) anions or promote the homolytic

production of toxic hydroxy (HO^1) and hydroperoxy (HOO^1) radicals.
These ideas are substantiated by the finding that haem, which
cleaves H_2O_2, and naphthoquinones which increase the levels of
H_2O_2 are lethal to T. brucei and T. cruzi in vitro (Meshnick et
al 1978; Boveris et al 1978). In T. brucei naphthoquinones are
thought to inhibit the co-enzyme Q factor in the unique terminal
electron transport system thus favouring the production of H_2O_2
whereas in T. cruzi they may promote the production of superoxide
anions and H_2O_2 which interact to produce toxic hydroxy (HO^1)
radicals, unfortunately naphthoquinones show little activity in
vivo due to poor pharmacokinetics. However another important
component of the cellular defence mechanism against H_2O_2 and free
radicals is believed to be glutathione (GSH): Cerami and his
collaborators (Arrick et al 1981) have recently confirmed this
and demonstrated that buthione sulphoxime (BSO) (a potent and
specific inhibitor of γ glutamylcysteine synthetase, the first
enzyme in the glutathione biosynthesis pathway), administered to
T. brucei infected mice results in a progressive decrease in
trypanosome GSH content and a fall in parasitaemia when blood
levels of the drug were maintained for 18 hrs. The large doses
of BSO required to cure mice preclude the therapeutic use of this
compound but the work opens up a new approach and indicates a
means by which a biochemical difference between parasite and host
may be therapeutically exploited. BSO appears to be entirely
non-toxic to mammalian cells and to date T. brucei is the only
organism known to be damaged by BSO - induced GSH depletion
(almost certainly due to the parasites inability to inactivate
self generated H_2O_2). As Arrick et al (1981) have indicated the
possibility that a practical therapy might be based on less
rapidly excreted inhibitors of GSH biosynthesis administered with
compounds, such as naphthoquinones, which increase the level of
intracellular peroxide is clearly attractive and should be
pursued. The mechanisms by which free radicals are scavenged by
parasitic protozoa have been little studied. Recent work (Docampo
et al 1981) suggests that the nitrofuran, nifurtimox (one of the
two drugs on the market for treatment of Chagas' disease) may act
by generation of toxic oxygen radicals. The stages of T. cruzi
and Leishmania sp. which develop intracellularly are known to
survive phagocytic killing mechanisms (one of which involves the
production of O_2^- and H_2O_2) and there is evidence (Meshnick and
Eaton, 1981) that Leishmania tropica does not fail to stimulate
the oxidative burst of the macrophage but evades the toxic
effects of O_2^- by the production of high levels of a superoxide
dismutase which differs from the host cell enzyme. Clearly the
mechanisms used by these parasites to neutralize free radicals
should be further investigated: novel therapeutic targets may
well be identified.

Amino Acids, Purines and Pyrimidines

Attempts to culture microorganisms in defined media often bring to light nutritional and metabolic idiosyncrasies: this proved to be the case with Trypanosoma brucei (Cross et al 1975). It was found that the amino acid L-threonine rapidly became depleted and subsequent work showed that it is cleaved by threonine dehydrogenase to form glycine and acetate the latter being a preferred source of 2C units for fatty acid synthesis even in the presence of exogenous acetate and a 10-fold molar excess of glucose (Klein and Linstead, 1976). The apparent importance of this pathway in trypanosomes compared to mammalian cells suggests that a search for inhibitors may prove profitable and is currently being pursued.

A number of workers have noted that the pathway of pyrimidine synthesis could be an attractive locus for chemo-therapy. Plasmodia, babesia and some kinetoplastid flagellates, in contrast to their hosts, are known to be dependent upon de novo synthesis and detailed studies of the enzymes involved are in progress in a number of laboratories (Gero and Coombs, 1980; Gutteridge et al 1979). A particularly interesting development from this area of research is the finding by Marr et al (1978) that Leishmania and T. cruzi metabolise allopurinol sequentially to aminopurinol mononucleotide which is incorporated into RNA in contrast to the pathway in man which involves conversion to oxipurinol and excretion. Allopurinol appears to be inactive in vivo probably due to the rapidity with which it is excreted, but it may prove possible to use this system as a model for synthesis of other antiprotozoal agents.

Cell Structures

In the course of adapting to life in the mammalian blood-stream the African trypanosomes have evolved an ingenious mechanism by which they evade the hosts immune response. Infection is characterized by a relapsing parasitaemia in which each recrudescence represents the appearance of a new antigenic type characterized by a distinct glycoprotein 'coat' overlying the cell surface membrane. This surface coat of variant specific antigen (VSA), which is present on developmental stages of the parasite found in the salivary gland of the vector (Glossina sp.) and in the bloodstream of the mammalian host but absent from the stages developing in the vector midgut, has attracted a great

deal of research effort in the last decade. The molecular basis
of antigenic variation has been clarified (Cross, 1978): the
surface coat consists of a single glycoprotein with a molecular
weight of about 55-65,000, glycoproteins from different
trypanosome variants differ in amino acid composition, conformational features and N-terminal amino acid sequences. It is
not known how many immunologically different surface glycoproteins
a single trypanosome can make but it is thought to be in excess
of 100. These findings raise many important questions: how are
the antigens synthesised? How is the synthesis controlled and
switched to a new VSA? How are the glycoproteins assembled and
attached to the cell surface? Space does not permit and it would
not be appropriate here to review in detail the spectacular
advances made in recent years towards answering these questions:
readers are referred to a comprehensive review by Turner (1982).
What is relevant to this discussion is the possibility that the
process of antigenic variation may involve mechanisms unique to
the parasites which could be potential chemotherapeutic targets.
There is already evidence that the process involves, as a first
step, gene duplication to produce an 'expression linked copy'
which is transposed to another region of the genome and modified
by replacement of the 3' end of the gene. The glycoprotein
precursor polypeptide produced from this gene undergoes post-
translational changes involving processing an N-terminal signal
peptide and two stages of glycosylation. A selective inhibitor
of any one of these stages could prove to be a potent chemotherapeutic agent acting not by destroying the parasite but by
allowing host defence mechanisms to control the infection. A
second possibility is that knowledge of the way VSA is assembled
and inserted into the cell membrane may suggest ways of disrupting
this association so exposing invariant antigens of the underlying
membrane to the hosts immune attack. Structural studies indicate
that different VSAs contain areas of homology at the C-terminal
end and these are believed to be involved in membrane binding.
This is a most promising area of research with, I believe, great
chemotherapeutic potential.

Another unique feature in the cell structure of all haemo-
flagellates which is being considered as a potential chemotherapeutic target is the pellicular microtubular network. The
role of these microtubules is not fully understood: it has been
suggested that they play an important role in morphogenesis
(reviewed by Vickerman and Preston, 1976) and their functional
integrity may be required for the control and maintenance of
membrane related physiological processes essential to the
parasites survival in the host. Drugs known to affect the state
of microtubule polymerization in other cell systems (eg
Vinblastine or Taxol, an experimental antitumour drug isolated

from the plant <u>Taxus brevifolia</u> and known to inhibit HeLa cell
replication) have been reported to inhibit trypanosome replication
(Baum <u>et al</u> 1981) and since preliminary comparative studies
(Lagnado - unpublished observations) have detected differences
between trypanosome and mammalian tubulins further study of this
system could be rewarding.

Parasite/Host Cell Interactions

It has long been known that intracellular development in
specific host cells is an obligatory stage in the development of
some parasitic protozoa but we are only just beginning to learn
something of the mechanisms by which such parasites identify and
penetrate these cells. Such knowledge could well be relevant to
the search for new control methods. For example, plasmodial
sporozoites rapidly leave the bloodstream to begin their pre-
erythrocytic cycle of development in the cytoplasm of hepatocytes;
there is doubt about whether they initially invade hepatocytes or
cells lining the sinusoids but clearly selective invasion of
liver cells implies there is a specific recognition mechanism.
Could infection be prevented by interfering with this mechanism?
Recent experiments using fluorescent lectins (Schulman <u>et al</u> 1980)
have shown that none of the major sugar moieties known to be
expressed on cell surfaces are exposed on the surface of
<u>Plasmodium berghei</u> sporozoites and treatment with enzymes known
to expose hidden lectin-binding sites in other cells was without
effect, however, when sporozoites were incubated in mouse serum
lectins specific for mannose and galactose were bound, implying
that serum components with these sugars as terminal residues had
become firmly attached to the sporozoites. The binding was
species specific, the rodent parasite <u>P. berghei</u> binding components from rodent but not primate serum and vice versa with
the primate parasite <u>P. knowlesi</u>. It has been suggested that the
serum components may be involved in the recognition of cells in
liver invaded by sporozoites since it is known that there are
mannose receptors on Kupffer cells and galactose receptors on
hepatocyte plasma membranes and circulating glycoproteins with
terminal galactose residues are bound and taken up by hepatocytes. Perhaps sporozoites exploit an existing system for uptake
of glycoproteins by liver cells, this hypothesis could provide an
explanation for some intriguing results obtained by Alving <u>et al</u>
(1979) who have shown that intravenous injection of liposomes
containing neutral glycolipids with terminal galactose residues
prevents the appearance of erythrocytic forms of <u>P. berghei</u> in
mice infected one day previously with sporozoites but did not
inhibit infection transmitted by injecting parasitised
erythrocytes. Are the liposomes interfering with sporozoite

entry into or development in hepatocytes? As Peters (1980) has
pointed out other explanations must be considered but this whole
area of research seems to have considerable potential for new
approaches to malaria control.

Intracellular Parasites and Drug Targetting

No discussion of new chemotherapeutic strategies in 1982
would be complete without mention of drug targetting. This topic
is discussed in detail in a later paper by Dr. Gregoriadis but we
agreed that I should mention briefly the way this approach is
being applied to protozoal diseases. The intracellular location
of some of these parasites during different stages of their life
cycles poses special problems for chemotherapy - the leishmania
are a case in point, within the mammalian host the parasites are
restricted almost exclusively to cells of the reticulo-endothelial
system - the parasites are found within a parasitophorous vacuole
where they resist lytic enzymes and free radicals introduced by
lysosome fusion. As mentioned earlier the visceral form of the
disease, caused by L. donovani and L. infantum developing mainly
in liver spleen and bone marrow, frequently fails to respond to
drug treatment, but the very location of the parasites in the
deep organs would seem to make them ideal targets for lysosomotropic agents and particularly liposomes. In general the use of
liposomes in chemotherapy suffers from the disadvantage that on
intravenous injection the vesicles are rapidly cleared by
phagocytic cells of liver and spleen but in the case of visceral
leishmaniasis this is a positive advantage and there have been
several reports of the enhanced activity of antimonial compounds
and other drugs incorporated into liposomes in the treatment of
L. donovani infections in mice or hamsters (reviewed by Peters,
1980): in some experiments liposome encapsulated sodium
stibogluconate was found to be 700 times as effective as the free
drug. The cutaneous form of leishmaniasis where parasites are
restricted to skin macrophages might not be expected to respond
so well to liposome entrapped drugs but Chance and New (1980)
have reported that they are more effective than free drug in
experimental infections in mice. Thus there is now every reason
to hope that preparations based on this principle will provide a
more effective and less toxic way of administering antimonials in
the treatment of the varied forms of this disease.

For the same reasons the hepatic stage of plasmodial
infections could be particularly susceptible to liposome entrapped
drugs. I have already discussed the interesting experiments of
Alving et al (1979) with liposomes containing neutral glycolipids with terminal galactose residues, which are active alone

94

(ie in the absence of an entrapped drug). The possibility of combining a known prophylactic antimalarial (primaquine, 6-methoxy-8-aminoquinoline, which acts predominantly on the exoerythrocytic stages of Plasmodia) with liposomes has been explored by Pirson et al (1980). They found that although primaquine in cholesterol-rich liposomes is no more effective than the free drug, it is considerably less toxic (the LD_{50} being increased 3.5 times) and this more favourable therapeutic index permits a single curative dose to be administered to sporozoite infected mice. These workers also report that the toxicity of primaquine can be reduced by covalent linkage of the amino acid leucine to the free amino group of the drug molecule. This derivative is stable in serum but is rapidly broken down by lysosomal enzymes to release free drug. The reduced toxicity of leucyl-primaquine permits administration of a single dose capable of producing 100% cure in experimental infections, the therapeutic index being increased from 1.5 for primaquine to 3.7 for leucyl-primaquine.

Unfortunately these approaches to the chemotherapy of intra-cellular infections are less likely to be effective against Chagas' disease. Amastigotes of Trypanosoma cruzi that are responsible for the chronic phase of infection which has proved so difficult to treat are not restricted to the phagocytic cells of the reticulo-endothelial system they also develop, for example, in cardiac muscle and other host cells which may not take up lysosomotropic drug complexes. There has been a preliminary report (Trouet et al 1976) that the veterinary drug ethidium bromide is more effective against T. cruzi infections in mice if it is administered as a complex with DNA but these experiments are difficult to interpret – the DNA-drug complex may be acting as a slow release formulation rather than being targetted to parasitized host cells.

NEW LEADS FROM CANCER CHEMOTHERAPY AND THE MODIFICATION OF EXISTING DRUGS

Ethidium bromide is one of a series of phenanthridine derivatives with trypanocidal activity which have been used to treat the disease in cattle for over thirty years. These drugs are known to be potent inhibitors of DNA synthesis acting by intercalation between adjacent base pairs of the DNA helix (reviewed by Newton, 1976). This knowledge led to the screening of other known inhibitors of DNA synthesis (eg antibiotics and anticancer drugs) for trypanocidal activity in standard mouse screens, but with singularly little success, however, some

95

investigators have also used in vitro screens and compounds have been found which although inactive in vivo possess a high in vitro activity. Until recently little effort has been made to investigate the reasons for such differences but the work of Williamson et al (1981) suggests that this could be a rewarding approach. They found that the antitumour drug daunorubicin is a potent trypanocide in vitro, it permanently abolishes the infectivity of African trypanosomes at nanomolar concentrations but is totally inactive against trypanosome infections in rodents. A study of the distribution of daunorubicin Trypanosoma rhodesiense infected mice showed that the drug was present in the plasma and was taken up by the trypanosomes but was not retained by them as the blood level of drug fell due to excretion. Since activity of drugs is often proportional to length of exposure as well as to concentration these workers have explored the possibility of modifying daunorubicin so as to increase and maintain drug levels in the plasma and, by exploiting the endocytic activity of trypanosomes, within the parasites. They found that covalent coupling of drug to protein (albumin and ferritin have been used) leads to retention of trypanocidal activity in vivo however, the nature of the coupling is all important, only those conjugates in which the drug is coupled to protein via a labile linkage are active in vivo suggesting that trypanocidal activity may depend upon drug being released intracellularly.

The possible value of drug/carrier conjugates and slow release formulations has not been fully explored in the treatment of protozoal infections: I believe it should be.

Relatively few of the very large number of compounds synthesised in the search for anticancer agents have been screened for activity against parasitic protozoa. This is an approach which is being actively encouraged by the UNDP/World Bank/WHO Special Programme. A very promising new lead which has recently emerged from the dual approach of seeking inhibitors of specific metabolic pathways in trypanosomes and screening existing anticancer drugs is an inhibitor of polyamine biosynthesis. The polyamines commonly found in animals and plants are putrescine, spermidine and spermine but bloodstream trypomastigotes are unusual in that they lack spermine. They synthesise putrescine and spermidine de novo from ornithine and methionine (Bacchi et al 1979). In mammalian cells polyamines are believed to act as stabilizers for nucleic acids (tRNA, ribosomes and DNA) and are thought to play an important role in cell division, dividing cells having elevated polyamine levels. In mammalian cells the rate controlling step in polyamine synthesis is thought to be that catalysed by ornithine decarboxylase (ODC) which has a high turnover rate and is very susceptible to external inducers. Because ODC induction and polyamine synthesis are associated with the onset of growth in all pro- and eukaryotic organisms studied it has been pointed out (Bacchi, 1981) that this enzyme is "a logical target for chemotherapy of disease states characterized by rapid cell proliferation". An analogue of ornithine, α-difluoromethyl-ornithine (DFMO) has been reported to inhibit the growth of various mammalian cells but is a compound of remarkably low toxicity (Seiler et al 1978) and is a specific enzyme activated inhibitor of ODC and hence of putrescine synthesis. These facts led Bacchi et al (1980) to test DFMO against T. brucei infections in mice: it was found that animals given the drug as a 1 or 2% solution in their drinking water were completely cured, parasites disappeared from the blood after five days treatment and when drug administration ceased after six days no relapses occurred over a two month period; uninfected mice inoculated with blood or brain suspension from cured animals remained uninfected. These encouraging results have led some field workers (perhaps prematurely) to treat some cases of late stage sleeping sickness with DFMO, favourable results have been reported but it is too early to conclude that this drug can cure such cases. Experiments with animal models for late stage infections suggest that relapses can occur after DFMO treatment.

CONCLUSION

It will be clear to you by now that this discussion of new strategies is more than slightly biased towards the African trypanosomes. Those of you who know my own research interests may not be too surprised, but, in fact, this bias is not solely a reflection of my own interests. In recent years the salivarian trypanosomes have caught the imagination of a new generation of cell biologists. As Turner (1982) has pointed out these organisms "seem almost to have been created to cater for the special interests of this new wave of biochemists and molecular biologists. So great is the trypanosome's potential for research on topics as diverse as mitochondrial gene expression, control of glycolysis, structure and function of membrane proteins and control of gene activity, that recently a special (EMBO, 1980) workshop was dedicated solely to introducing it to research workers as a model eukaryotic cell". The new leads for selective inhibitors now emerging from basic research on the biochemistry of trypanosomes and other protozoan parasites reflects the interest now being shown in these organisms by scientists from many disciplines and I am confident that major advances in the chemotherapy of the diseases they cause will result.

REFERENCES

Alving, C.R., Schneider, I., Swartz, G.M. and Steck, E.A. (1979). Sporozoite Induced Malaria: Therapeutic effects of glycolipids in liposomes. Science 205, 1142-1144.

Arrick, B.A., Griffith, O.W. and Cerami, A. (1981). Inhibition of Glutathione Synthesis as a Chemotherapeutic Strategy for Trypanosomiasis. J. Exp. Med., 153, 720-725.

Bacchi, C.J. (1981). Content, Synthesis and Function of Polyamines in Trypanosomatids: Relationship to Chemotherapy. J. Protozool., 28, 20-27.

Bacchi, C.J., Vergara, C., Garofalo, J., Lipschik, G.Y. and Hutner, S. (1979). Synthesis and Content of Polyamines in Bloodstream Trypanosoma brucei. J. Protozool., 26, 484-488.

Baker, J.R. (1982). The Biology of Parasitic Protozoa. Edward Arnold, London,

Baum, S.G., Wittner, M., Nadler, J.P., Horwitz, S.B., Dennis, J. E., Schiff, P.B. and Tanowitz, H.B. (1981). Taxol, a Microtubule Stabilizing Agent Blocks Replication of Trypanosoma cruzi. Proc. Natl. Acad. Sci., 78, 4571-4575.

Boveris, A., Docampo, R., Turrens, J.F., Stoppani, A.O.M. (1978). Effect of β-Lapachone on Superoxide Anion and Hygrogen Peroxide Production in Trypanosoma cruzi. Biochem. J., 175, 431-439.

Chance, M.L. and New, R.R. (1980). The Use of Lysosome Entrapped Drugs in the Treatment of Experimental Cutaneous and Visceral Leishmaniasis. In The Host-Invader Interplay. (ed. H. van den Bossche). Elsevier/North Holland, Amsterdam,

Clarkson, A.B. and Brohn, F.H. (1976). Trypanosomiasis: an Approach to Chemotherapy by the Inhibition of Carbohydrate Metabolism. Science 194, 204-206.

Clarkson, A.B., Grady, R.W., Grossman, S.A., McCallum, R.J. and Brohn, F.H. (1981). Trypanosoma brucei brucei: a Systematic Screeing for Alternatives to Salicylhydroxamic Acid - Glycerol Combination. Mol. Biochem. Parasit., 3, 271-291.

Cross, G.A.M. (1978). Antigenic Variation in Trypanosomes. Proc. Roy. Soc. Ser. B., 202, 55-72.

Cross, G.A.M., Klein, R.A. and Linstead, D.J. (1975). Utilization of Amino Acids by Trypanosoma brucei in Culture: L-threonine as a Precursor of Acetate. Parasitology 71, 311-326.

Evans, D.A. and Brown, R.C. (1973). m-Chlorobenzhydroxamic Acid - an Inhibitor of Cyanide - Insensitive Respiration in Trypanosoma brucei. J. Protozool., 20, 157-160.

Evans, D.A. and Holland, M.F. (1978). Effective Treatment of Trypanosoma vivax Infections with Salicylhydroxamic Acid (SHAM). Trans. Roy. Soc. Trop. Med. Hyg., 72, 203-204.

Evans, D.A., Brightman, C.J. and Holland, M.F. (1977). Salicyl-hydroxamic Acid/Glycerol in Experimental Trypanosomiasis. Lancet ii, 769.

Fairlamb, A.H., Opperdoes, F.R. and Borst, P. (1977). New Approach to Screening Drugs Against African Trypanosomiasis. Nature (London) 265, 270-271.

Fulton, J. and Spooner, J. (1956). Inhibition of the Respiration of Trypanosoma rhodesiense by Thiols. Biochem. J., 63, 475-481.

Gero, A.M. and Coombs, G.H. (1980). Orotate Phosphoribosyl-transferase and Orotidine.5'.Phosphate Decarboxylase in Two Parasitic Kinetoplastic Flagellates. FEBS Letters 118, 130-132.

Grant, P.T. and Sargent, J.R. (1960). Properties of L-α-Glycerophosphate and its Role in the Respiration of Trypanosoma rhodesiense. Biochem. J., 76, 229.

Gutteridge, W.E., Dave, D. and Richards, W.H.G. (1979). Conversion of Dehydro-orotate to Orotate in Parasitic Protozoa. Biochim. Biophys. Acta 582, 390-401.

Hammond, D.J. and Bowman, I.B.R. (1980). Trypanosoma brucei: The Effect of Glycerol on the Anaerobic Metabolism of Glucose. Mol. Bioch. Parasitol., 2, 63-75.

Klein, R.A. (1980). Principles in the Chemotherapy of Protozoan Disease. In Veterinary Medicine. (eds. A.T. Phillipson, L.W. Hall and W.R. Pritchard). Heinemann, London,

Klein, R.A. and Linstead, D.J. (1976). Threonine as a Preferred Source of 2-carbon Units for Lipid Synthesis in Trypanosoma brucei. Biochem. Soc. Trans., 4, 48-50.

Marr, J.J., Berens, R.L. and Nelson, D.J. (1978). Anti-trypanosomal Effect of Allopurinol: Conversion in vivo to Aminopyrazole Pyrimidine Nucleotides by Trypanosoma cruzi. Science 201, 1018–1020.

Meshnick, S.R., Blobstein, S.M., Grady, R.W. and Cerami, A. (1978). An Approach to the Development of New Drugs for African Trypanosomiasis. J. Exp. Med., 148, 569–579.

Meshnick, S.R., Chang, K.P. and Cerami, A. (1977). Heme Lysis of the Bloodstream Forms of Trypanosoma brucei. Biochem. Pharmacol., 26, 1923–1928.

Meshnick, S.R. and Eaton, J.W. (1981). Leishmanial Superoxide Dismutase: a Possible Target for Chemotherapy. BBRC 102, 970–976.

Newton, B.A. (1976). Antiprotozoal Drugs as Biochemical Probes. In Biochemistry of Parasites and Host–Parasite Relationships. (ed. H. van den Bossche). North Holland, Amsterdam,

Opperdoes, F.R. and Borst, P. (1977). Localization of nine Glycolytic Enzymes in a Microbody-like Organelle in Trypanosoma brucei: The Glycosome. FEBS Letters 80, 360–364.

Opperdoes, F.R., Borst, P. and Fonck, K. (1976). The potential Use of Inhibitors of Glycerol.3.Phosphate Oxidase for Chemotherapy of African Trypanosomes. FEBS Letters 62, 162–172.

Opperdoes, F.R., Borst, P. and Spits, H. (1977). Particle Bound Enzymes in the Bloodstream Form of Trypanosoma brucei. Europ. J. Biochem., 76, 21–28.

Peters, W. (1980). Therapy of Intracellular Parasitic Infections with Lysosomotropic Drugs. In The Host–Invader Interplay. (ed. H. van den Bossche). Elsevier/North Holland, Amsterdam,

Pirson, P., Steiger, R.F., Baurain, R., Masquelier, M. and Trouet, A. (1980). Antimalarial Activity of Liposomal Primaquine and Peptidic Derivatives of Primaquine. In The Host–Invader Interplay. (ed. H. van den Bossche). Elsevier/North Holland, Amsterdam,

Schulman, S., Oppenheim, J.D. and Vanderberg, J.P. (1980). Plasmodium berghei and Plasmodium knowlesi: Serum Binding to Sporozoites. Exp. Parasit., 49, 420–429.

Taylor, M.B., Berghausen, H., Heyworth, P., Messenger, N., Rees, L.J. and Gutteridge, W. (1980). Subcellular Localization of some

Glycolytic Enzymes in Parasitic Flagellate Protozoa. Int. J.
Biochem., 11, 117-120.

Trouet, A., Jadin, J.M. and van Hoof, F. (1976). Lysosomotropic
Chemotherapy in Protozoal Diseases. In Biochemistry of Parasites
and Host-Parasite Relationships. (ed. H. van den Bossche).
Elsevier/North Holland, Amsterdam,

Turner, M.J. (1982). Biochemistry of the Variant Specific
Glycoprotein of Salivarian Trypanosomes. Adv. Parasitol., 20,
69-153.

Vickerman, K. and Preston, T.M. (1976). Comparative Cell Biology
of the Kinetoplastid Flagellates. In Biology of the Kineto-
plastida. (eds. W.H.R. Lumsden and D.A. Evans). Academic Press,
London,

Visser, N. and Opperdoes, F.R. (1980). Glycolysis in
Trypanosoma brucei. Europ. J. Biochem., 103, 623-632.

von Brand, T. and Johnson, E.M. (1947). A comparative Study of
the Effect of Cyanide on the Respiration of some Trypanosomatidae.
J. Cell Comp. Physiol., 29, 33-49.

Williamson, J., Scott-Finnigan, T.J., Hardman, M.A. and Brown,
J.R. (1981). Trypanocidal Activity of Daunorubicin and Related
Compounds. Nature (London) 292, 466-467.

Anthelminthic chemotherapy

R E Howells

Department of Parasitology
Liverpool School of Tropical Medicine, Pembroke Place
Liverpool, L3 SQA, UK

The annual worldwide cost of parasitic disease in livestock
has been estimated at $6 billion, or to be equivalent to a loss of
at least 5 million metric tons of ruminant protein output. These
losses result from the increased mortality, reduced fertility and
impaired growth rate of diseased stock, together with the lowered
production of meat, milk, wool, fibre and leather (Kelly and Hall,
1979). Chemotherapy is essential to the control of these diseases
and an indication of its value to both the livestock and pharmaceutical industries can be obtained from the observation that in
1978 £15 million was spent on anthelminthics and their application
to cattle in England and Wales alone (Michel et al., 1981). In
tropical countries parasitic diseases of man also have great public
health and socio-economic importance. At least 200 million people
in Southeast Asia, South America and the Caribbean are believed to
be infected by schistosomes (Duke, 1978) and more than 250 million
by the lymphatic dwelling filarial worms Wuchereria bancrofti and
Brugia malayi (Sasa, 1976). A further 20 million people in
tropical Africa, the Yemen, Mexico, Central and South America are
infected by Onchocerca volvulus, the causative agent of river
blindness (Sasa, 1976). A majority of the population in many
countries of the tropics and subtropics also are infected by gastrointestinal nematodes, including Ascaris lumbricoides, the hookworms
Ancylostoma duodenale and Necator americanus, and the whipworm
Trichuris trichiura. Ascaris lumbricoides, alone, is thought to
infect over 700 million people, about 26% of the world population
(Muller, 1975). Amongst some ethnic groups and in some geographic
areas individual helminth diseases may achieve particular
significance, such as hydatid disease amongst the Turkana people
of Northern Kenya. Duke (1978) discussed the association of
parasitic disease and poverty in these countries and observed that,
as a result of poverty, medical anthelminthics do not provide an
economically attractive market for the pharmaceutical industry.

103

The major incentive for the industrially based development of new anthelminthics is therefore to be found in the veterinary field. To compensate for this situation the World Health Organisation has promoted a research programme aimed at combatting the six most important of the 'neglected' diseases of the tropics; these include two helminthiases, schistosomiasis and filariasis.

ANTHELMINTHIC AGENTS

The structures of some of the anthelminthics referred to in this paper are presented in Table 1. A survey of the older anthelminthic compounds was presented by Cavier and Hawking (1973) and Kelly et al. (1976) reviewed the history of the development of ruminant anthelminthics. Other recent reviews include those by Wagner and Duwel (1980) and Werbel and Worth (1980).

A prominent feature of anthelminthic chemotherapy during the past two decades has been the development of benzimidazole compounds with activity against nematodes, cestodes and trematodes. The first of the benzimidazole anthelminthics was thiabendazole and this was followed by a series of derivatives with differing properties. The activities of the benzimidazoles commercially available in 1977 were summarised by Coles (1977). Each of the benzimidazole anthelminthics has a high level of activity against most of the adult nematodes of the intestinal tract but the more recently developed benzimidazoles are of significance since they differ from thiabendazole in the degree of their activity against tissue parasites, such as lung worms, arrested larval nematodes, cestodes and liver flukes. The introduction of albendazole as a fasciolicide in the late 1970s, for example, was of particular importance in the USA since hexachloroethane which had previously been employed against fascioliasis in bovines had been removed from the US Food and Drug Administration's (FDA) list of approved animal drugs at a time when the occurrence and prevalence of Fasciola hepatica in cattle in the United States was increasing. Loyacano et al. (1980) and Bradley et al. (1981) described the effect of albendazole on Fasciola hepatica infections in calves. During a 250 day study period the body weight of albendazole treated calves increased by 43 lbs/head more than thiabendazole treated (control) animals and the liver condemnation rates on slaughter were 3% and 32% for the albendazole and thiabendazole groups, respectively (Loyacano et al., 1980). The efficacy against adult flukes of albendazole given as an oral drench, was 63.4%, 50.0% and 56.6% for dosages of 15.0, 10.0 and 7.5 mg/kg, respectively, but only at the highest dosage was there an effect against immature flukes (Bradley et al., 1981). The activity of albendazole against liver flukes, tapeworms, lung- and gastro-intestinal nematodes was described by Theodorides et al. (1976).

The numbers of inhibited fourth stage Ostertagia ostertagi in yearling beef cattle given fenbendazole orally at 5 mg/kg, were reduced by 47.6% with considerable variability being observed in individual animals (Williams et al., 1981a). Adult populations of all intestinal nematodes were reduced by 79.4% by the same drug treatment. Oxfendazole at 10 mg/kg was highly effective against adult nematodes in the intestine of horses and removed 83-88% and 97-99% of the fourth stage larvae of Strongylus vulgaris in the mesenteric arteries and S. edentatus in flank lesions, respectively. Early fifth stage S. vulgaris larvae were, however, less susceptible and the drug was without obvious effect against adult forms of the tapeworm Anoplocephala perfoliata.

An important feature of the benzimidazole anthelminthics is their potential for activity against zoonotic nematode infections of man such as Trichinella spiralis and Toxocara canis. A series of articles dealing with the effects of albendazole, febantel, fenbendazole, flubendazole, cambendazole, mebendazole, oxibendazole, parbendazole and other anthelminthics on T. spiralis are included in the Proceedings of the Fifth International Conference on Trichinellosis (Kim et al., 1981). In these Proceedings, Spaldonova (1981) showed that febantel (N-{2-[2,3-Bis-(methoxy-carbonyl)-guanidino]-5-(phenylthio)-phenyl}-2-methoxy-acetamid) was more effective than fenbendazole against encysted muscle larvae though fenbendazole is an active metabolite of febantel in vivo. In sheep both febantel and fenbendazole are rapidly and substantially converted to oxfendazole (Pritchard, 1982). Duwel (1981) showed that when fenbendazole was given in medicated feed over five days it was more effective than equivalent single daily doses. 100 ppm fenbendazole eliminated all pre-adult and adult intestinal stages, 200 ppm eliminated migrating stages but 500 ppm (0.05%) were required for effect upon the encysted muscle larvae. A similar pattern was observed by Thienpoint and Vanparijs (1981) in a well documented study of the effect of flubendazole against T. spiralis in pigs. All doses higher than 32 ppm were 100% effective against the intestinal and migrating larval stages but encysted larvae were more resistant; a dose of 125 ppm administered over 14 days was necessary for 100% effect on 3-5 week old cysts and an even higher dosage was required for elimination of older cysts.

Mebendazole and fenbendazole are effective against human enterobiasis (Bhandari and Singhi, 1980) and mebendazole has been successfully employed in human capillariasis (Van den Bossche, 1980). An extensive analysis of the activity of mebendazole, flubendazole and other benzimidazole derivatives against larval echinococcosis (hydatid disease) in man and animals was made by Schantz et al. (1982). Mebendazole or flubendazole treatment of patients infected with Echinococcus granulosus is followed by subjective improvement in most and evidence of regression of cysts in some, but in other patients cysts continue to grow or have been proven viable even after several months of high dose mebendazole therapy. E. multilocularis, the cause of alveolar hydatid disease, was not killed by treatment with the drugs but the progressive course of the disease appeared halted.

The development of a safe anthelminthic with activity against the adult stages of Onchocerca volvulus is one of the major goals of medical helminthology. Mebendazole has recently been shown by Rivas Alcala et al. (1981) and Awadzi et al. (1982) to possess a degree of activity in patients with onchocerciasis. Mebendazole at 2 g/day for 28 days or mebendazole at the same dosage plus levamisole (150 mg once weekly for five doses) caused a reduction in the number of skin microfilariae and embryogenesis had been interrupted in adult worms removed from patients at two months post drugging (Rivas Alcala et al., 1981). Mebendazole alone was also observed to inhibit temporarily embryogenesis in adult worms by Awadzi et al. (1982) but these workers found that reductions in the skin microfilarial densities were only achieved when mebendazole was given in combination with levamisole.

The marked differences in efficacy of the several benzimidazole anthelminthics against gastro-intestinal nematodes and tissue-dwelling parasites are due not only to differences in the vermicidal properties of the drugs per se but also to differences in the pharmacological properties and pharmacokinetic behaviour of the compounds. Studies with mebendazole have shown that in man and most other mammalian species, less than 10% of an orally administered dose is absorbed and the absorbed drug is rapidly metabolised; in man the half-life in normal individuals varying from 2.5-5.4 hr. The absorption of mebendazole was also dose-independent, a 20-fold increase in dosage resulting only in a 1.4-fold increase in the plasma level. The anthelminthic activity of all identified metabolites of mebendazole is also lower than that of the parent compound (see Schantz et al., 1982). These data have particular relevance to the therapy of hydatid disease. Plasma mebendazole levels above 73.7 ng/ml were associated with a significant decrease in the weight of hydatid cysts in animals but in patients who received mebendazole orally at 200 mg/day for three days (a level recommended for treatment of intestinal nematodes) the plasma level of the drug never exceeded 30 ng/ml. When patients received oral doses of 16 to 60 mg/kg/day no correlation was found between the dosage and the plasma mebendazole concentration, which varied widely between 4 and 575 ng/ml (median 40; n = 48). Flubendazole injected subcutaneously in jirds at 100 mg/kg conferred a residual filaricidal effect of between 9 and 12 weeks (Denham and Brandt, 1980) as a result of 'depot' formation at the injection site. Studies to obtain an improved injectable formulation of this anthelminthic are currently in progress.

Pharmacological profiles of albendazole and oxfendazole in sheep were reported by Marriner et al. (1980) and Shastri et al. (1980) respectively. Comparison of the pharmacokinetics of ^{14}C-fenbendazole with ^{3}H-thiabendazole, following intraruminal application to cattle, revealed that fenbendazole persists longer in the gut lumen and plasma than does thiabendazole because it is absorbed and recycled more slowly and is more extensively recycled to the intestinal tract. The area under the plasma concentration curve of fenbendazole in cattle is ten times greater than that of thiabendazole when related to the same dose (Prichard, 1982). The closure of the oesophageal groove in sheep was correlated with ruminal by-pass and changes in the pharmacokinetic behaviour and efficacy of oxfendazole (Prichard, 1980). Closure of the oesophageal groove resulted in by-pass of the rumen by the orally administered drug, which in turn led to a reduction in the area under the plasma concentration curve, an earlier peak plasma concentration and a reduction in efficacy against benzimidazole-resistant Haemonchus contortus.

A considerable body of evidence has now accumulated to identify helminth tubulin as a primary receptor for the anthelminthic benzimidazoles. Friedman and Platzer (1980) observed that the inhibition constants of mebendazole and fenbendazole for the polymerisation of bovine brain tubulin was 7.3×10^{-6}M and 1.7×10^{-5}M respectively. The corresponding values for mebendazole and flubendazole with Ascaris suum embryonic tubulin were 1.9×10^{-8}M and 6.5×10^{-8}M respectively. The inhibition of embryonic tubulin polymerisation was correlated with the activity of benzimidazoles against developing parasite embryoes (see Van den Bossche, 1980; Rivas Alcala et al., 1981; Awadzi et al., 1982). Intestinal tubulin from the adult Ascaris suum was also recognised as a target sensitive to mebendazole by Kohler and Bachmann (1980). In contrast to the Ki values obtained for mebendazole with Ascaris embryonic tubulin $(1.9 \times 10^{-8}$M) however, the Ki with intestinal tubulin was $4.2 \mp 0.4 \times 10^{-6}$M. The values obtained for pig brain tubulin $(8.0 \mp 0.9 \times 10^{-6}$M) by Kohler and Bachmann (1980) were similar to those obtained by Friedmann and Platzer (1980) for bovine brain tubulin $(7.3 \times 10^{-6}$M).

Kohler and Bachmann (1980) considered it doubtful whether the small difference in affinity of mammalian brain and the Ascaris intestinal tubulin could be responsible for the apparently selective activity of the drug against the parasite. Significant differences were found in the pharmacokinetic behaviour of the drug in the host and parasite, however, the drug being readily taken up by intact worms which were incapable of metabolising it to any significant extent within a 24 hr period of incubation. After the 24 hr incubation period in vitro the internal drug concentrations greatly exceeded those of the external medium.

Ultrastructural studies have identified the primary site of mebendazole action in the intestines of Ascaris suum and Syngamus trachea (Borgers et al., 1975) and of Ascaridia galli (Atkinson et al., 1980) as the organelles involved in the secretory mechanism of the intestinal cells; the drug-induced block in transport of secretory granules and in the movement of other subcellular organelles coinciding with the disappearance of cytoplasmic microtubules. Earlier suggestions that succinate dehydrogenase-fumarate reductase was a possible site of action for mebendazole, thiabendazole and cambendazole have been re-examined by several workers. Comley and Wright (1981) observed that a significant inhibition of fumarate reductase from Aspiculuris and Ascaris suum was obtained only by using $1 \times 10^{-3}M$ thiabendazole and that no inhibition occurred with $1 \times 10^{-4}M$ thiabendazole or cambendazole. The fumarate reductase from a thiabendazole-resistant Haemonchus contortus however, was shown to have a reduced sensitivity to thiabendazole and cambendazole (see Pritchard, 1982).

In the cysticerci of Taenia taeniaeformis and the hydatid cysts of E. granulosus mebendazole induces changes in the germinal membranes similar to those observed in the intestine of nematodes (see Schantz et al., 1982; Al-dabagh et al., 1981; Laclette et al., 1981). Mebendazole at $9.2 \times 10^{-3}M$ inhibited by 50% malate-induced phosphorylation in Ascaris mitochondria (Van den Bossche, 1976). The drug also decreased ATP synthesis in Moniezia expansa (Rahman and Bryant, 1977; Rahman et al., 1977) and a feature of benzimidazole action on both nematodes and cestodes is an apparent effect on glucose absorption (Van den Bossche, 1976; Rahman and Bryant, 1977; Duwel, 1977). A marked increase in the permeability of hydatid cysts to 3-0-methyl glucose followed exposure to $3.4 \times 10^{-6}M$ mebendazole in vitro for 12 hours (Reisin et al., 1980; quoted in Schantz et al., 1982).

Glucose utilisation was also inhibited in the filarial worm Brugia pahangi following drugging in vivo with flubendazole and mebendazole at 100 mg/kg (unpublished observation).

Yamamoto (1980) isolated and analysed genetically mutants of the fission yeast Schizosaccharomyces pombe which were resistant to thiabendazole and methyl-2-benzimidazole carbamate, both of which compounds are inhibitors of nuclear division in the parent yeast. Single mutations gave rise to both resistances, indicating a common target(s) for both drugs. Tuyl (1975) selected and identified three separate classes of thiabendazole-resistant mutants of Aspergillus nidulans, one of which was highly resistant and the map position of the resistant gene (ben A) was defined. Ben A was demonstrated by Sheir-Neiss et al. (1978) to be a structural gene for β-tubulin.

Other anthelminthics with a high level of efficacy against intestinal nematodes include levamisole, pyrantel, methyridine and bephenium hydroxynaphthoate. Discussion of these compounds can be found in Cavier and Hawking (1973) and an analysis of their mechanisms of activity, and of the pyrantel analogues, morantel and oxantel, was made by Van den Bossche (1980). Cabrera et al. (1980) and Sinniah and Sinniah (1981) described the effect of flubendazole, oxantel-pyrantel and mebendazole and of pyrantel pamoate, oxantel-pyrantel pamoate, levamisole and mebendazole on intestinal nematodes of man.

Levamisole, the L-isomer of DL-tetramisole has been employed as an anthelminthic for more than a decade. Recent interest in the compound has centred on its immunopotentiating properties (Symoens, 1980; Plowman, 1981) and apparent synergy when used with other anthelminthics. Bennet et al. (1980), for example, observed a potentiation of effect when mebendazole and levamisole were used together on sheep infected with benzimidazole-resistant Haemonchus contortus. An apparent synergistic effect of mebendazole and levamisole combinations against O. volvulus (Awadzi et al., 1982) has been previously noted. The toxicity of levamisole was however, significantly increased in pigs when levamisole was administered in combination with pyrantel tartrate (Hsu, 1981), supporting the hypothesis that nicotine-like compounds enhance levamisole toxicity. No reduction in the LD_{50} of levamisole was observed when co-administered with the organophosphate dichlorvos. Optomisation of the properties of levamisole were sought by Hogarth-Scott et al. (1980) and Forsyth and Wynne-Jones (1980) who determined that when injectable levamisole plus a polyvalent clostridial vaccine were tested in sheep the combined preparation resulted in a significantly heightened antibody response whilst the anthelminthic efficacy of levamisole was unimpaired. A useful account of parasite host interactions relative to levamisole was presented by Guerrero (1980).

Of the anthelminthics which have been developed in recent years hycanthone, oxamniquine, praziquantel and amoscanate possess high levels of efficacy against some or all species of schistosome infecting man. Hycanthone possesses activity against Schistosoma mansoni and S. haematobium and has been used for the treatment of approximately 1.2 million people (Dennis, 1978). Prata (1976) reviewing its usage in over 100,000 patients in Brazil, considered that it may be too toxic for such large scale use and much debate has centred on the toxicity and potential mutagenicity of hycanthone (Ong, 1978). Bueding and Batzinger (1979) considered various methods of reducing the mutagenic properties of the drug, including co-administration with erythromycin to eliminate the production of mutagenic metabolites by microorganisms. Five years investigation into possible genetic effects of hycanthone on mice were reported by Russell and Generoso (1982) however, who concluded that there is no basis for recommending that the use of hycanthone should cease.

The earlier information on the mode of action of hycanthone showed that though it is a non-competitive inhibitor of schistosomal acetylcholinesterase the mechanism of its therapeutic action could not be related to this capacity (Van den Bossche, 1980). It was also reported that the activity of hycanthone might be related to the displacement of acetylcholine from the acetylcholine receptor site in schistosomes (Hillman et al., 1978). Kim et al. (1981) found that hycanthone, but not praziquantel was a potent inhibitor of monoamine oxidases from worms and mouse liver. Mattoccia et al. (1981) presented data to indicate that inhibition of RNA synthesis, through inhibition of uridine incorporation, may be the mechanism of action of hycanthone.

A more recently developed schistosomicide, oxamniquine, is active against S. mansoni infections as a short course oral treatment. Structurally it resembles hycanthone in possessing an alkylaminoethyl amino group para to a hydroxymethyl group and is an inhibitor of schistosome acetylcholinesterase (Van den Bossche, 1980). Kilpatrick et al. (1981) summarised five years' experience in the treatment of S. mansoni infections in Egyptian patients with oxamniquine. Cure rates of 55% and 87% for children and adults respectively, in an uncomplicated group were obtained. 24 of 29 (83%) of patients with colonic polyposis were cured and each of 24 patients with hepatic decompensation due to S. mansoni infection were cured. It was concluded that oxamniquine results in a low cure rate in children but was safe and effective in adults. Kaye (1979) compared the pharmacokinetics of oxamniquine in patients in Brazil and several geographical regions of Africa and concluded that geographical differences in the dose response of oxamniquine are not due to pharmacogenetic differences in different ethnic groups but are more likely due to different susceptibilities of the various geographic strains of S. mansoni.

Amoscanate (C 9333 - 90/GCP 4540), 4-isothiocyanate-4'-nitro-phenyldiamine is an experimental schistosomicidal compound which possesses activity against each of the human species of schistosome together with a range of cestode and nematode parasites, including filarial worms (Striebel, 1976; Sen and Deb, 1981). The potential of these compounds was confirmed by clinical trials in man against hookworm infections and Ascaris lumbricoides, Trichuris trichiura and Enterobius vermicularis (Vaidya et al., 1977; Vakil et al., 1977; Doshi et al., 1977). Batzinger et al. (1979) reported that administration of amoscanate to uninfected Cebus apella and Macaca mulatta or to schistosome infected primates was followed by the appearance of mutagenic material in the urine. This mutagenic activity was eliminated by the co-administration

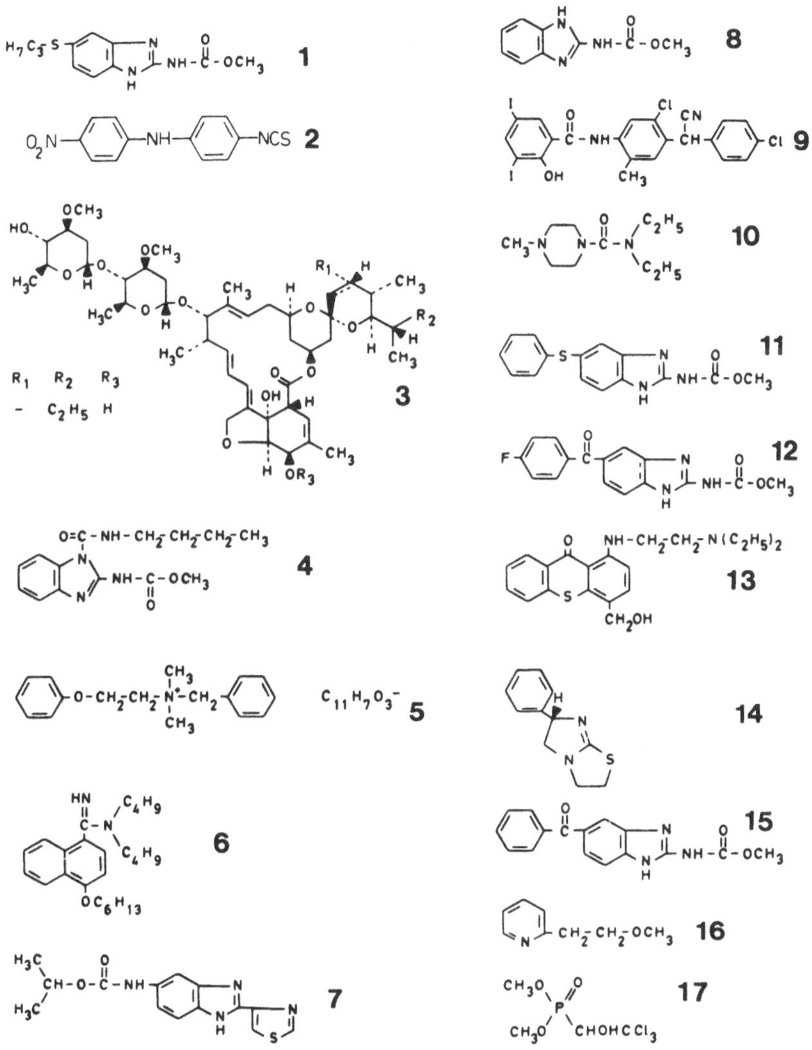

Figure 1 : The structure of some anthelminthic compounds

1 albendazole;   2 amoscanate;   3 avermectin B_{1a};   4 benomyl;
5 bephenium hydroxynaphthoate;   6 bunamide;   7 cambendazole;
8 carbendazin;   9 closantel;   10 diethylcarbamazine;
11 fenbendazole;   12 flubendazole;   13 hycanthone;   14 levamisole;
15 mebendazole;   16 methyridine;   17 metrifonate

Figure 1 continued..

18 morantel; 19 niclosamide; 20 nocodazole; 21 oxamniquine;
22 oxantel pamoate; 23 oxibendazole; 24 parbendazole;
25 piperazine; 26 praziquantel; 27 pyrantel pamoate;
28 rafoxanide; 29 Ro 11-3128; 30 suramin; 31 thiabendazole.

of erythromycin (as reported by Batzinger and Beuding (1979), for hycanthone). Voge and Bueding (1980) examined by scanning electron microscopy tegumental surface alterations in S. mansoni following the administration of subcurative doses of amoscanate.

A highly effective schistosomicidal compound, praziquantel, was introduced in 1975. This compound has activity against all three species of human schistosome and is also highly active against adult and larval cestodes (Gonnert and Andrews, 1977; Webbe and James, 1977; Thomas and Gonnert, 1977). Although this drug is without effect upon Fasciola hepatica it is active against other trematode infections of man including Opisthorchis viverrini (Ambroise-Thomas et al.,1981), Clonorchis and Opisthorchis (Horstmann et al., 1981; Loscher et al., 1981). Praziquantel was also effective against Diplostomum spathaceum in rainbow trout (Bylund and Sumari, 1981).

Ultrastructural studies of the surface of various cestode and trematode species after praziquantel treatment (Becker et al., 1980; Becker et al., 1981) have identified characteristic tegumental lesions which developed within five minutes of exposure to the drug. In a series of elegant studies on the mode of action of praziquantel, Fetterer, Bennett and their colleagues have shown that the sustained contracture of the musculature of adult male S. mansoni could be correlated with high internal Ca^{++} levels resulting from drug induced changes in the permeability of the parasite's muscle cells to Ca^{2+} (Fetterer et al., 1980; Wolde Mussie et al., 1982).

Other anthelminthics which have been identified as schisto-somicides include the benzodiazipines, clonazepam and Ro 11-3128 (Stohler, 1978). Preliminary work in South Africa suggested that Ro 11-3128 as a single oral dose of 0.2 to 0.3 mg/kg is effective against single and mixed infections of S. mansoni and S. haematobium (Baard et al., 1980). Bennett (1980) identified and described a low affinity benzodiazipine binding site in intact or homogenised male S. mansoni using [^{14}C] Ro 11-3128 and [^{3}H] clonazepam. Since Ro 11-3128 would produce an increase in worm muscle tension within 1-2 sec. and a rapid increase (within 15 sec.) in the influx of ^{45}Ca^{++} into male schistosomes (Pax et al., 1978) the binding site may be located on the epidermis of male schistosomes (Bennett, 1980).

Closantel is a recently developed salicylanilide anthelminthic which is highly effective against Fasciola hepatica, F. gigantica, blood sucking nematodes and the insect larval stages of Oestrus ovis, Dermatobia sp. and Hypoderma sp. (Theinpoint et al., from Van den Bossche, 1980). Van den Bossche (1980) reviewed earlier data that closantel in vitro and in vivo uncouples oxidative

113

phosphorylation. The anthelminthic specificity of this uncoupler is presumably associated with its pharmacokinetic properties, for although it uncoupled phosphyralation in both parasite and mammalian mitochondria in vitro, only parasite mitochondria were uncoupled in vivo. Kane et al. (1980) also studied the mode of action of closantel and reported that it increased mitochondrial permeability and uncoupled oxidative phosphorylation. A further novel fasciolicide is MK-401 (4-amino-6-trichloroethanyl 1,3-benzenesulfonamide). Ostlind et al. (1977) and Mrozik et al. (1977) described the anthelminthic properties of this compound which was active against Fasciola hepatica in sheep and cattle. The drug was shown to inhibit glucose utilisation and acetate and propionate formation in the flukes through inhibition of phosphoglycerate kinase and phosphoglyceromutase (Schulman and Valentine, 1980). In a further study (Schulman et al., 1982), the effect was described of MK-401 and analogues with different substituents at the 6 position of the aromatic ring, on purified F. hepatica phosphoglycerate kinase. A good correlation was found between the activity and the size of the substituent at the 6 position. Mammalian and yeast phosphoglycerate kinases are known to be bilobed enzymes with a nucleotide cleft which undergo a large conformational change when phosphoglycerate binds and it was speculated that if the fluke enzyme has a similar structure the large substituent on the 6 position of MK-401 (or analogues) could block the conformational change and inhibit the enzyme.

One of the most remarkable developments in anthelminthic chemotherapy during recent years has been the discovery by workers at the Merck Sharp and Dohme Research Laboratories of the avermectins. The first report of these compounds was made in 1978 and an interesting account of their discovery and properties has been given by Campbell (1981). The avermectins are glycosidic derivatives of macrocyclic lactones which are produced by a species of actinomycete, Streptomyces avermitilis, isolated from soil in Japan. They do not possess the antibacterial properties associated with 'macrolide' antibiotics but when activity was first detected and the activeingredient added to animal feed, it was found that it was active against Nematospiroides dubius in mice at one part per million (a level significantly lower than can be employed with other anthelminthics). The compounds were isolated by solvent extraction of the mycelia of S. avermitilis and first separated into four major (a) components by a series of silica gel chromatograms. From each of these (a) components, 5-10% of a minor (b) homologue could be separated by reverse phase high-performance liquid chromatography. There are thus eight avermectins, designated A_{1a} to B_{2b}. Of these various compounds, avermectin B_{1a}, 22, 23-dihydro-avermectin, was selected for commercial development as 'ivermectin'. Ivermectin contains at least 80% 22,23-dihydro-avermectin B_{1a}, which has a secondary butyl substituent at the 25 position, and not more than 20% of B_{1b}

which has an isopropyl substituent at the 25 position. It was
rapidly shown that in addition to possessing remarkable
anthelminthic activity at dosage levels as low as 10 μg/kg, they
were particularly active against parasites and stages difficult
to treat by some anthelminthics; fourth stage larval nematodes,
lungworms, and drug-resistant parasite strains. Additionally,
the avermectins were active against arthropod ectoparasites, mites
and ticks. A comparison of thiabendazole, levamisole hydrochloride
and the major natural avermectins against Trichostrongylus
colubriformis in gerbils by Ostlind and Cifelli (1981) showed that
85% and 100% of the worm burdens were removed by thiabendazole
and levamisole at 200 and 6.25 mg/kg respectively. Avermectin
B_{1a} and B_{2a} removed 100% of the worms at 0.0312 mg/kg. Ivermectin
has been shown active against fourth stage Strongylus vulgaris
(Slocombe and McCraw, 1981) and a wide range of other nematodes
(Craig and Kunde, 1981) of ponies; against the swine kidney
worm Stephanurus dentatus (Stewart et al., 1981a) as well as five
other genera of pig nematodes and the hog louse Haematopinus suis
(Stewart et al., 1981b). Benz and Ernst (1981a, b) Lyons et al.
(1981) and Williams et al. (1981b) have described the efficacy of
ivermectin against cattle nematodes.

In dogs infected with Dirofilaria immitis avermectin B_{1a} was
effective against microfilariae and against the developing tissue
stages, but not the adult forms of this filariid (Campbell and
Blair, 1981). The avermectins were also inactive against encysted
muscle forms of T. spiralis in laboratory animals (see Campbell,
1981).

The activity of the avermectins against nematode and arthropod
parasites has been related to the property of the compounds to
act as agonists of Y-aminobutyric acid (GABA) in both parasite
groups. In nematodes GABA is an inhibitory neuro-transmitter
involved in sending signals from the inhibitory interneurons to the
motor neurons whereas in arthropods it acts at the junction between
the motor neuron and the muscle cell. In both situations the
effect of the avermectin is thought to be mediated through
stimulation of release of GABA at the synapse which in turn results
in the opening of Cl-channels in the post junction membrane. The
result of the opening of the Cl-channels is a decrease in membrane
resistance and membrane hyperpolarisation, the motor neuron then
being unable to transmit impulses to the muscle. The failure of
avermectin to act on trematodes and cestodes can be correlated
with the apparent failure of these parasites to use GABA as a
neurotransmitter. There is also considerable evidence that GABA
is a major inhibitory neurotransmitter in the vertebrate central
nervous system and avermectins possess muscle relaxant effects in
rats (Williams and Yarborough, 1979). Pong and Wang (1982)
demonstrated that in vitro the number of post synaptic receptors

in rat brain membranes can be increased by avermectin when a functioning chloride ion channel is also present and that this effect may lead to an opening of chloride ion channels, a decrease in membrane resistance and membrane hyperpolarisation. Avermectin also stimulated benzodiazepine binding to rat brain membranes and solubilised receptor complex (Pong et al., 1981).

In this selective account of the more novel anthelminthics no mention has been given to many older, yet currently used anthelminthic compounds such as the organophosphates: metrifonate, a cheap yet effective agent against Schistosoma haematobium infections of man; suramin, which remains the only curative agent for O. volvulus infections; diethylcarbamazine, the drug of choice for treatment of lymphatic filariasis; piperazine, bephenium, hydroxynaphthoate, niridazole or the antimonial schistosomicides, details of which can be found in Cavier and Hawking (1973).

DRUG RESISTANCE IN HELMINTH PARASITES

An unwelcome development in the field of helminth chemotherapy particularly amongst nematodes of veterinary importance, has been the emergence of drug resistance. Extensive reviews of anthelminthic resistance in animal helminths by Kelly and Hall (1979). Prichard et al. (1980), examined the many aspects of the problem in farm animals and discussed the control of resistant parasites. The most widespread resistance occurs to benzimidazole compounds and a wide level of cross-resistance occurs within the class (Prichard et al., 1980; Prichard, 1982). Benzimidazole-resistant parasites have been reported from North and South America, Europe, South Africa, Australia and New Zealand. In Australia they already pose a serious problem, many parasite strains possessing a high level of benzimidazole resistance, cross resistance to several other classes of anthelminthics also occurring in some instances (Green et al., 1981). The mechanisms of resistance to benzimidazoles were discussed by Prichard (1982). Differences in benzimidazole uptake by sensitive and resistance parasites have been described but, by analogy with studies on hypersensitive, normal and benzimidazole resistant strains of Aspergillus nidulans, it is possible that tubulin from benzimidazole resistant nematodes may show an altered drug-binding constant. It has also been shown that inhibition of fumarate reductase is less pronounced in benzimidazole resistant than sensitive parasites (see Prichard et al., 1980). Subjection of benzimidazole strains of Haemonchus contortus and Ostertagia spp. to selection pressure over five laboratory generations with the recommended dose rates of cambendazole, oxfendazole or morantel resulted in a larger residual worm burden after treatment at the fifth generation, with both benzimidazoles. There was however, no change in response to morantel (Hall et al., 1981).

116

Levamisole resistance has also been described for several species of sheep, cattle and goat nematodes. Resistance to levamisole confers resistance to the morantel, oxantel, pyrantel group of drugs for, although differing chemically, they all act as cholinergic agonists at the level of the ganglion. The genetics of levamisole resistance was studied in the free-living nematode Caenorhabditis elegans (Lewis et al., 1980), the most resistant mutants of which might also lack pharmacologically functional acetylcholine receptors.

In the human helminthiases, drug resistance is a well reported phenomenon only in Schistosoma mansoni and with the drugs hycanthone and oxamniquine (see Kelly and Hall, 1979; Araujo et al., 1980). Such resistance may reflect variation in the hycanthone/oxamniquine base-line sensitivity levels of different geographic isolates of S. mansoni but resistance has also been developed experimentally by Bueding and others. An attempt to induce resistance to oxamniquine, hycanthone and praziquantel in S. mansoni in mice by continuous exposure to drug release from subcutaneous depots and by subcurative dosing by conventional routes of administration revealed that when four successive parasite generations were exposed to oxamniquine and hycanthone by either regimen the level of drug tolerance was increased. No similar effect was observed with praziquantel (Dr. I. Marshall, personal communication). Goven et al. (1980) described an apparent organophosphate resistance in the monogenetic trematode Gyrodactylus elegans on goldfish.

No resistance has yet been described to the avermectins.

DEVELOPMENTS IN THE DELIVERY OF ANTHELMINTHICS

Amongst the earliest attempts to develop novel methods of delivering anthelminthics to large population groups was the use of diethylcarbamazine-medicated cooking salt in the treatment of lymphatic filariasis (see Cavier and Hawking, 1973). A large number of studies have subsequently been employed with this medicated salt. More recently a further innovation in DEC administration was introduced by Langham et al. (1978) who applied DEC topically on patients with Onchocerca volvulus infections. The method of application appeared, on further examination, to offer no benefit over oral DEC since it gave no amelioration of the Mazzotti reaction. Phenothiazine-medicated salt licks have been employed in the control of ruminant helminthiases (Kelly and Hall, 1979).

Powers (1965) observed that antimony dimercapto succinate or piperazine hydrochloride in silicone rubber implants reduced the numbers of S. mansoni in mice. Collins (1974) later described the experimental use of silicone rubber capsules to provide a sustained release and microfilaricidal effect of the organophosphate famphur in Litomosoides carinii infected jirds. Olanoff et al. (1980) utilised similar devices to study the release and effect of niridazole in mice infected with S. mansoni and Marshall (1982a, b) examined the schistosomicidal effect of oxamniquine, praziquantel and of a thiophene derivative, and the cestodicidal effect of praziquantel, respectively, using silicone rubber drug mixture implants.

Guerrero et al. (1980) observed that an intraruminal sustained release bolus containing mebendazole protected lambs against experimental infection with several nematode species for up to seven weeks though levamisole containing bolus preparations were less effective. Anderson et al. (1980) and Le Jambre et al. (1981) showed that prolonged administration of oxfendazole to sheep by intraruminal controlled release capsules was found to be effective against both susceptible and thiabendazole resistant Haemonchus contortus and Ostertagia circumcincta and a thiabendazole resistant strain of Trichostrongylus colubriformis. The latter strain also showed cross resistance to oxfendazole at a dose rate of 5 mg/kg. Manger and Brewer (1980) described a slow release device for use in ruminants and obtained 12 weeks effect against sheep strongyles with a device containing morantel citrate. The only sustained release antihelminthic device which has been marketed for veterinary use however, is the morantel release bolus (Paratect bolus; Pfizer). Useful accounts of the application of the morantel bolus include Jones (1981) and Bliss et al. (1982). Administration of the bolus into the rumen of calves immediately before turnout onto spring pasture in May substantially reduced the level of pasture contamination with infective larvae later in the season and there was a 71% reduction in worm burdens acquired over the entire grazing season (Armour et al., 1981).

CONCLUSIONS

The advances which have been made in anthelminthic chemotherapy over recent years have resulted in the availability of drugs with a high level of efficacy against most of the helminths of veterinary and medical importance. There is still however, an outstanding need for better and safer drugs for use in the treatment of human filariasis and onchocerciasis and in the therapy of hydatid disease. An important consideration in medical helminthiases must also be the development of low cost drugs.

In veterinary helminthiases drug resistance poses a serious problem in some geographic areas and it is probable that resistance will attain increasing importance as the dependence on and use of anthelminthics increases. The economic importance of the ruminant helminthic infections, in particular, will however ensure a continued effort on the part of the pharmaceutical industry to identify new anthelminthics. It is to be hoped that the increasing knowledge of parasite biochemistry and physiology will facilitate the search for new drugs but the recent discovery of the avermectins emphasises the necessity for maintaining empirical screening programmes. In addition to novel agents, much potential benefit may be derived from improving the use of existing anthelminthics, such as through sustained release preparations and the use of mixtures of compounds with synergistic properties. The control of both veterinary and human worm diseases however, does not depend upon chemotherapy alone. The soil and water-borne infections of man have largely disappeared from the developed countries as a result of improved hygiene and the provision of adequate water supply and sewage removal systems. The improvement of sanitation and health education of man in the developing countries of the tropics will play an equally important part in disease control in helminth disease control. The control of veterinary helminthiases also depends upon complex control programmes which involve grazing and pasture management, nutritional supplementation and vaccination as well as chemotherapy (Kelly and Hall, 1979). The majority of such veterinary control schemes however have been developed in and for temperate climates and much remains to be learnt of control schemes appropriate to the tropics, where in a considerable number of countries the problems have not even been identified (Griffiths, 1978).

REFERENCES

Al-dabagh, M. A., Al-moslih, M. I., Verheyen, A., Shafik, M. A., Al-janabi, T. A., Al-rawas, A. Y., Ismail, M. A., Fawzi, A. H., Al-ani, M. S. and Rassam, S. (1981). The effect of mebendazole on sheep hydatid cysts as demonstrated by electron microscopy. J. Parasit., 67, 709-712.

Ambroise-Thomas, P., Goullier, A., Bonnet-Eumard, J. and Fournet, J. (1981). Treatment of Far-Eastern liver fascioliasis with praziquantel. Preliminary results in 30 patients. Nouvelle Press Medicale, 10, 427.

Anderson, N., Laby, R. H., Prichard, R. K. and Hennessy, D. (1980). Controlled release of anthelmintic drugs: a new concept for prevention of helminthosis in sheep. Res. Vet. Sci., 29, 333-341.

Araujo, N., Katz, N., Dias, E. P., and Souza, C. P. de (1980). Susceptibility to chemotherapeutic agents of strains of Schistosoma mansoni isolated from treated and untreated patients. Am. J. trop. Med. Hyg., 29, 890-894.

119

Armour, J., Bairden, K., Duncan, J. L., Jones, R. M. and Bliss, D. H. (1981). Studies on the control of bovine ostertagiasis using a morantel sustained release bolus. Vet. Record, 108, 532-535.

Atkinson, C., Newsam, R. J. and Gull, K. (1980). Influence of the antimicrotubule agent, mebendazole, on the secretory activity of intestinal cells of Ascaridia galli. Protoplasma, 105, 69-76.

Awadzi, K., Schulz-Key, H., Howells, R. E., Haddock, D. R. W. and Gilles, H. M. (1982). The chemotherapy of onchocerciasis, VIII. Levamisole and its combination with the benzimidazoles. Ann. trop. Med. Parasit. (in press).

Baard, A. P., Sommers, de K., Honiball, P. J., Fourie, E. D. and Du Toit, L. E. (1980). Ro-11-3128, a novel benzodiazepine schistosomicide: results in human schistosomiasis. In Current Chemotherapy and Infectious Disease, Volume 2. (eds. J. D. Nelson and C. Grassi). American Society for Microbiology, Washington DC.

Batzinger, R. P., Bueding, E., Crawford, K. and Bruce, J. (1979). Prevention of the mutagenic activation of an antischistosomal isothiocyanate in primates by an antibiotic. Environmental Mutagenesis, 1, 353-360.

Becker, B., Melhorn, H., Andrews, P. and Thomas, H. (1981). Ultrastructural investigations on the effect of praziquantel on the tegument of five species of cestodes. Z. Parasit., 64, 257-270.

Becker, B., Melhorn, H., Andrews, P., Thomas, H. and Eckert, J. (1980). Light and electron microscopic studies on the effect of praziquantel on Schistosoma mansoni, Dicrocoelium deudriticum and Fasciola hepatica (trematoda) in vitro. Z. Parasit., 63, 113-128.

Bennet, E. M., Behm, C., Bryant, C. and Chevis, R. A. F. (1980). Synergistic action of mebendazole and levamisole in the treatment of a benzimidazole-resistant Haemonchus contortus in sheep. Vet. Parasit., 7, 207-214.

Bennett, J. L. (1980). Characteristics of antischistosomal benzodiazepine binding sites in Schistosoma mansoni. J. Parasit., 66, 742-747.

Benz, G. W. and Ernst, J. V. (1981a). Anthelminthic efficacy of 22,23-dihydroavermectin B, against gastrointestinal nematodes in calves. Am. J. Vet. Res., 42, 1409-1411.

Benz, G. W. and Ernst, J. V. (1981b). Anthelminthic efficacy of ivermectin against immature gastrointestinal and pulmonary nematodes of calves. Am. J. Vet. Res., 42, 2097-2098.

Bhandari, B. and Singhi, A. (1980). Fenbendazole (Hoe 881) in enterobiasis. Trans. R. Soc. trop. Med. Hyg., 74, 691.

Bliss, D. H., Jones, R. M. and Conder, D. R. (1982). Epidemiology and control of gastrointestinal parasitism in lactating, grazing adult dairy cows using a morantel sustained release bolus. Vet. Record, 110, 141-144.

Borgers, M., De Nollin, S., De Brabander, M. and Thienpoint, D. (1975). Influence of the anthelminthic mebendazole on microtubules and intracellular organelle movement in nematode intestinal cells. Am. J. Vet. Res., 36, 1153-1166.

Bradley, R. E., Randell, W. F. and Armstrong, D. A. (1981). Anthelminthic efficacy of Albendazole in calves with naturally acquired Fasciola hepatica infections. Am. J. Vet. Res., 42, 1062.

Bueding, E. and Batzinger, R. P. (1979). New approaches towards the development of safer schistosomicidal drugs. In Advances in Pharmacology and Therapeutics, Volume 10. Chemotherapy. (ed. M. Adolphe). Pergamon Press, Oxford.

Bylund, G. and Sumari, O. (1981). Laboratory tests with Droncit against diplostomiasis in rainbow trout, Salmo gairdneri Richardson. J. Fish Dis., 4, 259-264.

Cabrera, B. D., Valdez, E. V. and Go, T. G. (1980). Clinical trials of broad spectrum anthelmintics against soil-transmitted helminthiasis. SE Asian J. Trop. Med. Pub. Hlth, 11, 502-506.

Campbell, W. C. (1981). An introduction to avermectins. New Zealand Vet. J., 29, 174-178.

Campbell, W. C. and Blair, L. S. (1981) The avermectins: a new family of compounds with activity against Dirofilaria immitis. In Proceedings Heartworm Symposium '80. Vet. Med. Publishing Co., Bonner Springs, Kansas.

Cavier, R. and Hawking, F. (eds.) (1973). Chemotherapy of Helminthiasis, Vol. I. Pergamon Press, Oxford

Coles, G. C. (1977). The biochemical mode of action of some modern anthelmintics. Pestic. Sci., 8, 536-543.

Collins, R. C. (1974). Implant chemotherapy of experimental filariasis. Am. J. trop. Med. Hyg., 23, 880-883.

Comley, J. C. W. and Wright, D. J. (1981). Succinate dehydrogenase and fumarate eductase activity in Aspiculuris tetraptera and Ascaris

suum and the effect of the anthelminthics cambendazole,
thiabendazole and levamisole. Int. J. Parasit., 11, 79-84.

Craig, T. M. and Kunde, J. M. (1981). Controlled evaluation of
ivermectin in Shetland ponies. Am. J. Vet.Res ., 42, 1422.

Denham, D. A. and Brandt, E. (1980). Chemoprophylactic activity of
flubendazole against adult Brugia pahangi transplanted into the
peritoneal cavity of jirds. J. Parasit., 66, 933-934.

Dennis, E. W. (1978). Global status of hycanthone: a review.
In Proceedings of the International Conference on Schistosomiasis,
Cairo, October 1975 Volume 1. (ed. A. Abdallah). Ministry of
Health, Cairo.

Doshi, J. C., Vaidya, A. B., Sen, H. G., Mankodi, N. A., Nair, C.N.
and Grewal, R. S. (1977). Clinical trials of a new anthelmintic,
4-isothiocyanato-4-nitrodiphenylamine (C9333-Go/GCP4540) for the
cure of hookworm infection. Am. J. trop. Med. Hyg., 26, 636-639.

Duke, B. O. L. (1978). The relevance of parasitology to human
welfare today - medical aspects. In Symposium of the British
Society of Parasitology, Vol. 16. (ed. A. E. R. Taylor and
R. Muller) Blackwell Scientific Publications, Oxford.

Duwel, D. (1977). Fenbendazole II. Biological properties and
activity. Pestic. Sci., 8, 550-555.

Duwel, D. (1981). Trichinellosis: successful treatment with
fenbendazole. In Trichinellosis (eds. C. W. Kim, E. J.
Ruitenburg, J. S. Teppema). Reedbooks, Chertsey.

Fetterer, R. H., Pax, R. A., Thompson, D., Bricker, C. and
Bennett, J. L. (1980). Praziquantel: mode of its antischistosomal
action. In Host Invader Interplay (ed. H. Van den Bossche),
Elsevier North Holland Biomedical Press, Amsterdam.

Forsyth, B. A. and Wynne-Jones, N. (1980). Levamisole vaccine
combinations. 2. Retained anthelmintic efficacy. Australian
Vet. J., 56, 292-295.

Friedman, P. A. and Platzer, E. G. (1980). Interaction of
anthelmintic benzimidazoles with Ascaris suum embryonic tubulin.
Biochem. Biophys. Acta., 630, 271-278.

Gonnert, R. and Andrews, P. (1977). Praziquantel, a new broad
spectrum antischistosomal agent. Z. Parasit., 52, 129-150.

Goven, B. A., Gilbert, J. P. and Gratzek, J. B. (1980). Apparent drug resistance to the organophosphate dimethyl (2,2,2-trichloro-1-hydroxyethyl) phosphonate by monogenetic trematodes. J. Wildlife Dis., 16, 343-346.

Green, P. E., Forsyth, B. A., Rowan, K. J. and Payne, G. (1981). The isolation of a field strain of Haemonchus contortus in Queensland showing multiple anthelminthic resistance. Australian Vet. J., 57, 79-84.

Griffiths, R. B. (1978). The relevance of parasitology to human welfare today - veterinary aspects. In Symposia of the British Society of Parasitology, Volume 16. (eds. A. E. R. Taylor and R. Muller) Blackwell Scientific Publications, Oxford.

Guerrero, J. (1980). Parasite host interactions relative to levamisole. J. Am. Vet. Med. Ass., 176, 1163-1165.

Hall, C. A., Kelly, J. D., Whitlock, H. V., Martin, I. C. A. McDonnell, P. A. and Gunawan, M. (1981). Five generations of selection with benzimidazole and non-benzimidazole anthelmintics against benzimidazole resistant strains of Haemonchus contortus and Ostertagia spp. in sheep. Res. Vet. Sci., 30, 138-142.

Hillman, G. R., Senft, A. W., Gibler, W. B. (1978). The mode of action of hycanthone revisited. J. Parasit., 64, 754-756.

Hogarth-Scott, R. S., Liardet, D. M. and Morris, P. J. (1980). Levamisole vaccine combinations. 1. Heightened antibody response. Australian Vet. J., 56, 285-291.

Horstmann, R. D., Feldheim, W., Feldmeier, H. and Dietrich, M. (1981). High efficacy of praziquantel in the treatment of 22 patients with Clonorchis-Opisthorchis infections. Tropenmed. Parasit., 32, 157-160.

Hsu, W. H. (1981). Drug interactions of levamisole with pyrantel tartrate and dichlorvos in pigs. Am. J. Vet. Res., 42, 1912-1914.

Jones, R. M. (1981). A field study of the morantel sustained release bolus in the seasonal control of parasitic gastroenteritis in grazing calves. Vet. Parasit., 8, 237-251.

Kane, H. J., Behm, C. A., and Bryant, C. (1980). Metabolic studies on the new fasciolicidal drug, closantel. Molec. Biochem. Parasit., 1, 347-355.

Kaye, B. (1979). Clinical experiences with, and pharmacokinetics of, oxamniquine. Part II. In Advances in Pharmacology and

Therapeutics, Volume 10. Chemotherapy. (ed. M. Adolphe). Pergamon Press, Oxford.

Kelly, J. D. and Hall, C. A. (1979). Resistance of animal helminths to anthelminthics. Adv. Pharm. Chem., 16, 89-128

Kelly, J. D., Gordon, H. McL. and Whitlock, H. V. (1976). Anthelminthics for sheep: historical perspectives, classification /usage, problem areas and future prospects. NSW Vet. Proc., 12, 18-31.

Kilpatrick, M. E., Farid, Z., Bassily, S., El-Masry, N. A., Trabobi, B. and Watten, R. H. (1981). Treatment of Schistosoma mansoni with oxamniquine - five years experience. Am. J. trop. Med. Hyg., 30, 1219-1222.

Kim, R. A., Lukacs, J., Tanaka, R. D. and MacInnis, A. J. (1981). Effects of hycanthone and praziquantel on monoamine oxidase and cholinesterases in Schistosoma mansoni. J. Parasit., 67, 20-23.

Kim, W. C., Ruitenburg, E. J. and Teppema, J. S. (eds.) (1981). Trichinellosis. Reedbooks, Chertsey.

Kohler, P. and Bachmann, R. (1980). The possible mode of action of mebendazole in Ascaris suum. In Host Invader Interplay. (ed. H. Van den Bossche). Elsevier/North Holland Biomedical Press, Amsterdam.

Laclette, J. P., Merchant, M. T., Wilms, K. and Canedo, L. (1981). Paracrystalline bundles of large tubules, induced in vitro by mebendazole in Cysticercus cellulosae. Parasitology, 83, 513-519.

Langham, M. E., Traub, Z. D., and Richardson, R. (1978). A transepidermal chemotherapy of onchocerciasis. Tropenmed. Parasit., 29, 156-162.

Le Jambre, L. F., Prichard, P. K., Hennessy, D. R. and Laby, R. H. (1981). Efficiency of oxfendazole administered as a single dose or in a controlled release capsule against benzimidazole-resistant Haemonchus contortus, Osterlagia circumcincta and Trichostrongylus colubriformis. Res. Vet. Sci., 31, 289-294.

Lewis, J. A., Wu, C. H., Berg, H. and Levine, J. H. (1980). The genetics of levamisole resistance in the nematode Caenorhabditis elegans. Genetics, 95, 905-928.

Loscher, T., Nothdurft, H. D., Prufer, L., Vonsonnenburg, F. and Lang, W. (1981). Praziquantel inclonorchiasis and opisthorchiasis Tropenmed. Parasit., 32, 234-236.

Loyacano, A. F., Malone, J. B. Jr., Pontif, J. and Nipper, W. A. (1980). A new weapon against liver flukes. Louisiana Agriculture, 23, 22-23.

Lyons, E. T., Tolliver, S. C., Drudge, J. H. and La Bore, D. E. (1981). Ivermectin: controlled test of anthelminthic activity in dairy calves with emphasis on Dictyocaulus viviparus. Am. J. Vet. Res., 42, 1225-1227.

Manger, B. R. and Brewer, M. D. (1980). Control of sheep roundworms with a long-acting ruminal device. In Proceedings of the Third European Multicolloquium of Parasitology, September 1980, Cambridge.

Marriner, S., Galbraith, E. A. and Bogan, J. A. (1980). Determination of the anthelminthic levamisole in plasma and gastrointestinal fluids by high performance liquid chromatography. The Analyst, 105, 993-995.

Marshall, I. (1982a). The activity of drug/silicone rubber mixtures against Schistosoma mansoni in laboratory mice. Ann. trop. Med. Parasit., 76, 113-114.

Marshall, I. (1982b). The effects of sustained-release praziquantel on the survival of Hymenolepis nana in laboratory mice. Ann. trop. Med. Parasit., 75, 115-116.

Mattoccia, L.P., Lelli, A. and Cioli, D. (1981). Effect of hycanthone on Schistosoma mansoni macromolecular synthesis in vitro. Molec. Biochem. Parasit., 2, 295-307.

Michel, J. F., Latham, J. O., Church, B. M. and Leech, P. K. (1981). Use of anthelminthics for cattle in England and Wales during 1978. Vet. Record., 108, 252-258.

Mrozik, H., Bochis, R. J., Eskola, P., Matzuk, A., Waksmunski, F.S., Olen, L. E., Schartzkopf, G., Grodski, A., Linn, B. O., Lusi, A., Wu, M. T., Shunk, C. H., Peterson, L. H., Milkowski, J. D., Hoff, D. R., Kulsa, P., Ostlind, D. A., Campbell, W. C., Riek, R. F. and Harmon, R. E. (1977). 4-amino-6-(trichloroethenyl)-1, 3,-benzenesulfonamide, a new potent fasciolicide. J. Med. Chem., 20, 1225-1227.

Muller, R. (1975). Worms and Disease - A Manual of Medical Helminthology. Heinemann Medical Books Ltd., London.

Olanoff, L. S., Mahmoud, A. A. F. and Anderson, J. M. (1980). Sustained release of niridazole from silicone rubber implants for the treatment of Schistosoma mansoni infections. Am. J. trop. Med. Hyg., 29, 71-73.

Ong, T. M. (1978). Genetic activities of hycanthone and some other antischistosomal drugs. Mutat. Res., 55, 43-70.

Ostlind, D. A. and Cifelli, S. (1981). Efficacy of thiabendazole, levamisolehydrochloride and the major natural avermectins against Trichostrongylus-Colubriformis in the gerbil (Meriones unguiculatus). Res. Vet. Sci., 31, 255-256.

Ostlind, D. A., Campbell, W. C., Riek, R. F., Baylis, P., Cifelli, S., Hartman, R. K., Lang, R. K., Bulter, R. W., Morozik, H., Bochis, R. J., Eskola, P., Matzuk, A., Wakmunski, F. S., Olen, L. E., Schwartzkopf, G., Grodski, A., Linn, B. O., Lusi, A. Wu, M. T., Shunk, C. H., Peterson, L. H., Milkowski, J. D., Hoff, D. R., Kulsa, P. and Harmon, R. E. (1977). The efficacy of 4-amino-6-trichlorocthemyl-1,3-benzenesulfonamide against liver fluke in sheep and cattle. Br. Vet. J., 133, 211-214.

Pax, R., Bennett, J. L. and Fetterer, R. (1978). A benzodiazepine derivative and praziquantel: effects on musculature of Schistosoma mansoni and Schistosoma japonicum. Naunyn-Schmiedeburg's Arch. Pharmacol., 304, 309-315.

Plowman, P. N. (1981). Levamisole: forerunner immunopotentiator. Trends Pharmacol. Sci., 2, vi.

Pong, Sheng-Shung and Wang, Ching Chung (1982). Avermectin B_{12} modulation of y-aminobutyric acid receptors in rat brain membranes. J. Neurochem., 38, 375-379.

Pong, S-S., Dettaven, R. and Wang, C. C. (1981). Stimulation of benzodiazepine binding to rat brain membranes and solubilised receptor complex by avermectin B_{1a} and y-aminobutyric acid. Biochim. Biophys. Acta, 646, 143-150.

Powers, K. G. (1965). The use of silicone rubber implants for the sustained release of antimalarial and antischistosomal agents. J. Parasit., 51, 53.

Prata, A. (1976). Experience in Brazil with the use of available schistosomicides in mass treatment campaigns. Rev. Soc. Brasil. Med. Trop., 10, 355-360.

Prichard, R. K. (1980). Host influences on the efficacy of benzimidazole anthelminthics. In Host Invader Interplay (ed. H. Van den Bossche). Elsevier/North Holland Biomedical Press, Amsterdam.

Prichard, R. K. (1982). Nuclear techniques in the study of resistance to antiparasitic agents. (in press).

Prichard, R. K., Hall, C. A., Kelly, J. D., Martin, I. C. A. and Donald, A. D. (1980). The problem of anthelminthic resistance in nematodes. Australian Vet. J., 56, 239-250.

Rahman, M. S. and Bryant, C. (1977). Studies of regulatory metabolism in Moniezia expansa: effects of cambendazole and mebendazole. Int. J. Parasit., 7, 403-409.

Rahman, M. S., Cornish, R. A., Chevis, R. A. F. and Bryant, C. (1977). Metabolic changes in some helminths from sheep treated with mebendazole. New Zealand Vet. J., 25, 79-83.

Rivas-Alcala, A. R., Greene, B. M., Taylor, H. R., Dominguy-Vazquez, A., Ruvalcaba-Macias, A. M., Lugo-Pfeiffer, C., Mackenzie, C. D. and Beltran, H. (1981). Chemotherapy of onchocerciasis: a controlled comparison of mebendazole, levamisole and diethylcarbamazine. Lancet, II, 485.

Russell, W. L. and Generoso, W. M. (1982). Investigations for transmitted genetic effects of hycanthone in mice. Helminth Abst., Ser. A., 51.

Sasa, M. (1976). Human Filariasis. University of Tokyo Press, Tokyo.

Schantz, P. M., Van den Bossche, H. and Eckert, J. (1982). Chemotherapy for larval echinococcosis in animals and man: a report of a workshop. Z. Parasit., 67, 5-26.

Schulman, M. D. and Valentino, D. (1980). Studies on the mechanism of action of 4-amino-6-trichloroethenyl-1,3-benzene-disulphonamide against Fasciola hepatica: effects on glycolysis in vitro. Expl Parasit., 49, 206-215.

Schulman, M. D., Ostlind, D. A. and Valentino, D. (1982). Mechanism of action of MK-401 against Fasciola hepatica: inhibition of phosphoglycerate kinase. Molec. Biochem. Parasit., 5, 133-145.

Sen, H. G. and Deb., B. N. (1981). Anthelminthic efficacy of amoscanate (C9333-Go/CGP4540) against various infections in rodents, dogs and monkeys. Am. J. trop. Med. Hyg., 30, 992-998.

Shastri, S., Moroszczak, E., Prichard, R. K., Parekh, P. Nguyen, T. H., Hennessey, D. R., Schiltz, R. (1980). Relationship among particle size distribution, dissolution profile, plasma values, and anthelmintic efficacy of oxfendazole. Am. J. Vet. Res., 41, 2095-2101.

Sheir-Neiss, G., Lai, M. H. and Morris, N. R. (1978). Identification of a gene for β-tubulin in Aspergillus nidulans. Cell, 15, 639-647.

Sinniah, B. and Sinniah, D. (1981). The anthelminthic effects of pyrantel pamoate, orantel-pyrantel pamoate, levamisole and mebendazole in the treatment of intestinal nematodes. Ann. trop. Med. Parasit., 75, 315-321.

Slocombe, J. O. D. and McGraw, B. M. (1981). Controlled tests of invermectin against migrating Strongylus vulgaris in ponies. Am. J. Vet. Res., 42, 1050-1051.

Spaldonova, R. (1981). Efficacy of febantel on Trichinella spiralis larvae in white mice. In Trichinellosis (eds. C. W. Kim, E. J. Ruitenburg, J. S. Teppema). Reedbooks, Chertsey.

Stewart, T. B., Marti, O. G. and Hale, O. M. (1981a). Efficacy of ivermectin against five genera of swinenematodes and the hog louse. Am. J. Vet. Res., 42, 1425-1426.

Stewart, T. B., Marti, O. G. and McCormick, W. C. (1981b). Efficacy of ivermectin against the swine kidney worm, Stephanurus dentatus. Am. J. Vet. Res., 42, 1427-1428.

Stohler, H. R. (1978). A novel schistosomacidal compound. Abstr. Cong. Chemotherapy, September 1977, Zurich, Switzerland.

Streibel, H. P. (1976). 4-isothiocyanate-4'-nitrodiphenylamine (C9333/CGP4540), an anthelminthic with an unusual spectrum of activity against intestinal nematodes, filariae and schistosomes. Experientia, 32, 457-458.

Symoens, J. (1980). Prospects for immunotherapy of 'parasitic' diseases. In Host Invader Interplay (ed. H. Van den Bossche). Elsevier/North Holland Biomedical Press, Amsterdam.

Theodorides, V. W., Gyurick, R. S. and Kingsbury, W. D. (1976). Anthelminthic activity of albendazole against liver flukes, tapeworms, lung and gastrointestinal roundsworms. Experientia, 32, 702-703.

Thienpoint, D. and Vanparijs, O. (1981). Prophylactic and curative action of flubendazole against experimental trichinellosis in pigs. In Trichinellosis (eds. W. C. Kim, E. J. Ruitenburg, Teppema, J.S.) Reedbooks, Chertsey.

Thomas, H. and Gonnert, R. (1977). The efficacy of praziquantel against cestodes in animals. Z. Parasit., 52, 117-127.

Tuyl, J. M. van (1975). Genetic aspects of acquired resistance to benomyl and thiabendazole in a number of fungi. Med. Fac. Landbouww Rijksuniv. Gent., 40, 691-697.

Vaidya, A. B., Sen, H. G., Mankodi, N. A., Paul, T. and Sheth, U.K. (1977). Phase 1 tolerability and searching dose studies with 4-isothiocyanato-4-nitrodiphenylamine (C9333-Go/GCP4540) a new anthelminthic. Br. J. Clin. Pharmacol., 4, 463-467.

Vakil, B. J., Dalal, N. J., Shah, P. N., Koti, S. T., Mankodi, N.A., Sen, H. G. and Vaidya, A. B. (1977). Clinical evaluation of a new anthelminthic - C9333-Go/CGP4540 in human hookworm infection. Trans. R. Soc. trop. Med. Hyg., 71, 247-250.

Van den Bossche, H. (1976). The molecular basis of anthelminthic action. In Biochemistry of Parasites and Host-Parasite Relationships. (ed. H. Van den Bossche). Elsevier/North Holland Biomedical Press, Amsterdam.

Van den Bossche, H. (1980). Peculiar targets in anthelminthic chemotherapy. Biochem. Pharm., 29, 1981-1990.

Voge, M. and Bueding, E. (1980). Schistosoma mansoni: tegumental surface alterations induced by subcurative doses of the schistosomicide amoscanate. Expl Parasit., 50, 251-259.

Wagner, W. H. and Duwel, D. (1980). Parasitology and therapy of tropical helminth infections. Immunitat und Infektion, 8, 64-74.

Webbe, G. and James, C. (1977). A comparison of the susceptibility to praziquantel of Schistosoma haematobium, S. japonicum, S. mansoni, S. intercalatum and S. matthei in hamsters. Z. Parasit., 52, 169-177.

Werbel, L.M. and Worth, D. F. (1980). Antiparasitic agents. In Annual Reports in Medicinal Chemistry, Volume 15. Academic Press, New York.

Williams, J. C., Knox, J. W., Baumann, B. A., Snider, T. G. and Hoerner, T. J. (1981a). Further studies on the efficacy of fenbendazole against inhibited larvae of Ostertagia ostertagi. Vet. Record., 108, 228-230.

Williams, J. C., Knox, J. W., Baumann, B. A., Snider, T. G., Kimball, M. G. and Hoerner, T. J. (1981b). Efficacy of ivermectin against inhibited larvae of Ostertagia ostertagi. Am. J. Vet. Res., 42, 2077-2080.

Williams, M. and Yarborough, G. (1979). Enhancement of the in vitro binding and some of the pharmacological properties of diazepam by a novel anthelminthic agent, avermectin B_{1a}. Eur. J. Pharmacol., 56, 273-276.

Wolde Mussie, E., Van de Waa, J., Pax, R. A., Fetterer, R. and Bennett, J. L. (1982). Schistosoma mansoni: calcium efflux and effects of calcium-free media on responses of the adult male musculature to praziquantel and other agents inducing contraction. Expl Parasit., 53, 270-278.

Yamamoto, M. (1980). Genetic analysis of resistant mutants to amitotic benzimidazole compounds in schizosaccharomyces-pombe. Molec. Gen. Genetics, 180, 231.

Major problems in cancer chemotherapy

Professor K Hellmann

Cancer Chemotherapy Department
Imperial Cancer Research Fund, P.O. Box 123
Lincolns Inn Fields, London WC2A 3PX, UK
and
Westminster Hospital, London, SW1

Cancer is a complex anarchic condition which results in much patient variation and is therefore difficult to classify except in loose anatomical and general terms. As a consequence, clinical trials of cancer treatment present considerable problems and interpretation is fraught with difficulties.

At present there are some 30 or so proven anti-cancer drugs but of these not more than half a dozen are in regular wide spread use. They vary from highly toxic compounds such as the anticancer antibiotic, adriamycin, producing regressions in a variety of malignancies to relatively innocuous hormonal substances such as tamoxifen with limited application in one particular cancer.

A vast number of compounds, probably in excess of 750,000, have been examined world wide for their anti-cancer activity but no specific antitumour compound has emerged. It is not surprising then that the first and most important problem of cancer chemotherapy is the discovery of some specific anticancer compounds. This process may be speeded up by the development of models with greater relevance than those currently available. The wide spread use of transplanted mouse tumours, although difficult to relate to any cancer in man may be of use if they could identify a specific anticancer agent, since it must be presumed that the development and progress of the ultimate malignant state is no different in the mouse than in man. The process of developing specific anticancer agents could also be helped by identification of the physico-chemical determinants of the malignant state.

Although it is unlikely that a cancer penicillin has been missed it is not difficult to believe that a cancer insulin might have slipped through the net. Moreover, although unlikely it is still possible that a cancer penicillin might have been missed simply because the degree of antitumour action of any drug depends on the complex integration of the pharmaco-kinetics of the drug and the cell kinetics of the tumour against which it is used.

Because it is not possible at present to describe the cancer state in therapeutically exploitable physico-chemical terms it is unavoidable that so-called random screening will have to continue for the foreseeable future. The current yield of this screening operation is not particularly high. At the National Cancer Institute of the United States the rate is about 1 investigational new drug in every 10,000 compounds examined.

A further developmental problem is that it could well be that the screens always select the same type of compounds. This is due to the fact that all efforts at finding anticancer drugs have been directed towards only one of the pathological features of the malignant state, namely that of uncontrolled proliferation. This in turn is due to the relatively easy way this pathological feature can be quantified and it also corresponds with most laboratory scientists' vision of what cancer is, namely a mass of uncontrolled prolif-erating cells. To be fair most clinical scientists also believed until quite recently that uncontrolled proliferation had to be the prime target since it seemed inherently impossible to reproduce the other anarchic characteristics of malignant tumours those of invasion, dissemination and metastasis formation which together form the crux of the clinical problem. It certainly seemed unlikely that these other pathological characteristics could be reproduced in such a way as to permit them to become quantitative and thus be used in laboratory tests.

Much interest is currently focussed on _in vitro_ systems, and they clearly confine themselves to analysis of proliferation as the chief malignant characteristic. It must of course be true that if one compound would emerge that could specifically prevent proliferation much would be solved, but pharmacokinetic and pharmaco-dynamic problems would still make it difficult for such substances to operate fully even if they were highly specific, particularly in patients with advanced tumours. The value of _in vitro_ tests for new or established drugs may lie much more in the elimination of ineffective drugs than in identification of effective drugs and thus patients might therefore be spared treatment with sub-stances which are unlikely to benefit them.

There have been attempts to produce a sensitivity test much along the lines of the bacterial sensitivity test systems for many years. First attempts were made as long ago as 1911 when Murphy and Sturm implanted a suspension of human tumour cells onto the chorio-allantoic membrane of the chick embryo with the purpose of allowing them to test substances directly on the patient's tumour. More recently using other systems, particularly in soft agar, many attempts have been made to grow human tumour stem cells as test systems for drugs. While in theory such systems sound attract-ive and plausible they have formidable technical problems to overcome before they could be confidently recommended as predictors of patients' responses to cancer chemotherapy. Not only do patients' tumour cells often fail to grow at all, but where there is growth it is not certain what type of cells have grown. The crucial test of reimplantation of the cells which

have grown _in vitro_ cannot of course be done and there
is some suspicion that most of the cells could be fibro-
blasts and not tumour cells at all.   Moreover, even if
they are tumour cells they may be the rapidly proliferating cells which are usually very sensitive to a
variety of anticancer drugs and therefore present much
less of a clinical problem.   The corollary is that
tumour cells that do not grow are the real problem and
that therefore the relevance of the _in vitro_ tests to
the question of identifying new drugs or more particularly drugs for the individual cancer patient is
questionable.

There are also technical complications as far as
the application of the drugs is concerned.   In most
in vitro tests the drugs are applied either for a very
short period of 1 hour or left in contact with the
cells for 24 or more hours.   A one hour exposure is
certainly unsatisfactory for phase specific compounds
since they will only be able to affect that fraction
(which may be quite small) of the total cells that
happen to be in the phase for which the compound is
specific.   If on the other hand the drugs are left in
the _in vitro_ medium for long periods of time, they may
undergo hydrolysis or other changes and will therefore
not reflect the concentrations or the substances to
which the tumours in the patient will be exposed.

In addition to all these difficulties there are
always the problems of drug metabolism _in vivo_ in the
process of which the real active agent may be formed
and which of course would not be tested when drugs are
applied directly to tumour cells.

It is also necessary to consider the general
problems of access to solid tumours which are completely
different from those of nicely dispersed tumour cells.
It is possible to summarise these problems in terms of
5 hurdles which any effective antitumour drug must
overcome.   These 5 hurdles are that the drug has to
be the right drug, delivered to the right cells in the

right concentration at the right time and for the right length of time. It must meet and overcome all of these hurdles at the same time if it is to be successful in producing a re sponse. The in vitro systems would (at best) only provide guidance for the first of these hurdles.

Even greater difficulties have in the past been encountered in the search for an adequate model for the other malignant characteristics of invasion, dissemination and metastasis formation and therefore almost no effort has been made to find substances which will interfere with these processes. One reason that is often advanced for inactivity in this area is that when patients are first diagnosed as having cancer they may already have clinically apparent metastases and/or micrometastases that may only reveal themselves at a later stage and there would therefore be little point in giving drugs to prevent a process that has already occurred. If however clinicians could be certain that no further metastases would develop, it would be possible to deal with those metastases that are present in the same way as multiple primary tumours, namely by local treatment. This would most certainly present a challenging task for surgery and radiotherapy.

Because of the anticipated difficulty in finding a useful model for metastasis it was for a long time thought that the only practical way of achieving this goal would be by the intravenous injection of tumour cells into animals, but this has raised many objections from pathologists and there is therefore considerable doubt about the validity of conclusions based on such a model.

It was only the development of the Lewis lung carcinoma system which showed for the first time that it was possible to have a spontaneously metastasizing transplantable tumour system which reproducibly, consistently and uniformly metastasized to the same

anatomical site at about the same time in all inoculated
animals and that could be used as a reasonably hard and
fast base line for observing the influence of a variety
of substances on this system.   Several compounds have
been shown to influence metastases formation in this
tumour without affecting the growth of the primary
carcinoma, but the problems of testing such substances
for antimetastatic activity in man is complex.

One reason for the complexity is that in most
tumours it is not possible to gauge accurately how much
clonogenic tumour is left after treatment.   Although
diagnostic imaging has become increasingly sophisticated,
tumours of less than 2cm are difficult to find by non-
invasive techniques.   Even if they are found it is not
possible to deduce much about their clonogenic ability
and repeat scans may not be able to differentiate a
progressive tumour from one whose cells have simply
enlarged in size, but not in number or where fluid
changes may have caused changes in size.   It is also
possible for the outer rim of the tumour to enlarge by
proliferation while the inner zone undergoes necrosis
at rates which cannot be determined, but which could
result in more, less or the same number of clonogenic
cells remaining.   It is also extremely difficult to be
certain how many subclinical micrometastases are already
present when the patient first receives antimetastatic
treatment.   As a result of these difficulties any trial
of antimetastatic compounds will take a long time to
evaluate.   This must mean that any compound to be
evaluated will have to be given for a long period of
time and it must therefore be sufficiently safe and
specific to permit this.

Clinical trials which take a long time to evaluate
also have built-in difficulties, since much can change
during the time of treatment.   Very few tumours are
suitable therefore for evaluation of antimetastatic
compounds.   Of all the tumours perhaps the most
suitable would be oat cell carcinoma of the bronchus
which usually metastasizes rapidly.   Treatment is

largely confined to chemotherapy or chemotherapy and irradiation, but despite any form of treatment available at present most patients die of disseminated disease within a year. Testing an antimetastatic compound in this condition has however to face the additional problem that oat cell carcinoma of the bronchus frequently spreads to the brain and any potential antimetastatic must therefore be capable of passing the blood-brain barrier, something of which most antitumour agents are not capable. There is however the hope and some evidence that even if an antimetastatic compound is not able to prevent metastases formation in the usual sites to which a tumour spreads it may change the sites at which the metastases occur and that this may permit the metastases to be more easily treated by localised or systemic treatment.

Alteration of the pattern of dissemination as a result of treatment has been observed in soft tissue sarcomas and colorectal cancer. It can be the result of regrowth delay following treatment for a sufficiently long period of time to allow metastases to develop in unusual sites, whereas previously patients might not have lived long enough to display this pattern. Soft tissue sarcomas often grow and disseminate rapidly, but hardly ever to the brain. When these tumours are treated with CyVADIC (cyclophosphamide, vincristine, adriamycin and DTIC) regressions may occur and time to recurrence may be increased, but survival is not, partly because a different pattern of metastases such as brain metastases may appear.

This change of metastases pattern has also been observed in an adjuvant trial of razoxane in colorectal cancer. The effect could be important in at least two ways, not only as has already been mentioned because the metastases might become more amenable to local or systemic treatment, but also because the disseminating cells might be kept circulating for a longer period within the lymphatic or blood stream thereby reducing both viable numbers and the virulence of the disseminating cells that can develop into metastases. The possibility that this might be correct has also been shown in a trial in which patients with circulating malignant cells were followed after their colonic tumour resection for at least 10 years. Those patients who pre-operatively had circulating tumour cells had a much longer recurrence free interval than those who had no circulating tumour cells. It seems possible that in this trial the circulating malignant cells were circulating because they were unable to implant, whereas in patients who had no circulating cells, malignant cells were able to leave the blood stream and invade organs. It will be necessary how-ever to repeat this trial with a closer and more detailed follow-up before any conclusions of substance can be drawn.

If little has been done on preventing metastases formation even less has been done on preventing invasion of adjacent tissues which is usually required before dissemination can take place. Mareel and his colleagues are now however attempting to validate a model which they have produced and which may be of im-portance in identifying drugs that could have anti-invasive effect.

Previous attempts to prevent dissemination of tumour cells at operation and reduce metastases were based on the belief that if metastases could not be demonstrated immediately before operation then sub-sequent metastases arose from tumour cells disseminated at operation. Clearly it cannot be a good idea to disseminate tumour cells at any time, but the major clinical problem of metastases appears to be that many micrometastases are already present at the time of or before operation and efforts aimed at preventing operative dissemination as a means to increasing re-currence free interval are therefore unlikely to succeed.

Another major problem, but hardly a surprising one, results from the non-selective inhibition of cell replication by the anticancer drugs. This results in predictable toxicity on normal proliferating cells, such as bone marrow, gastrointestinal mucosa, lymphoid tissue and gonadal tissues. In addition to these general toxic effects most agents have chronic and individual side-effects which may include neurological, pulmonary, cardiac, hepatic, renal and skin toxicities. Attempts are therefore being made at the present time not only by the time honoured method of analogue synthesis, but by more specific pharmacological actions, to reduce the dose-limiting toxicities of the anticancer drugs while maintaining their antitumour activity. Many of these attempts at reduction of toxicity and some of the attempts at increasing activity without increasing toxicity could be regarded as attempts at pharmacological response modification to yield a better therapeutic index. Some of the efforts have been demonstrated in model systems, but very few have shown any benefit as yet in clinical trials.

In view of the problems which have been pointed out in this short review, it is not altogether surprising that there is a marked contrast between the relatively sophisticated experimental attempts to find new anticancer drugs and the clinical trials which attempt to evaluate them. Phase II trials in particular, many of which are completely uninterpretable are subjected to statistical analyses which attempt to compare groups which are not comparable. Since not all the prognostic factors for any given tumour can be fully determined and even if they can be cannot be allowed for because of the large number of patients that might then be required, it is difficult to have adequately balanced comparative groups to permit statistics to be performed. It is doubtful whether merely increasing the size of a clinical trial population will overcome these difficulties and provide reliable statistical analysis. Large heterogeneous populations cannot be unscrambled merely by statistical devices. This results in contradictory

139

results on the rare occasions on which the results are
repeated.

Not only is there a problem then with adequately
comparable groups there is also a considerable difficulty in interpreting the end point of a trial, i.e.
the response.   This may be size of tumour, patient
survival or recurrence free interval.   Changes in
these parameters may depend on factors that are not
quantifiable, e.g. the degree of tumour stroma formation, extent of tumour oedema, vigour of antibiotic
treatment for intercurrent infection and administration
of other drugs that may have an influence on the anti-
cancer treatment of the trial.   Because of all these
difficulties the value of large multicenter trials
even if randomized and controlled are doubtful except
to confirm what has been found in smaller trials.

In view of all these difficulties it is surprising
that cancer chemotherapy has made the progress it un-
doubtedly has and particularly over the last ten years.

Chemotherapy of anaerobic bacteria

A T Willis

Public Health Laboratory, Luton
and
Luton and Dunstable Hospital, Luton, LU4 0DZ, UK

INTRODUCTION

Anaerobic bacteria cause a variety of disease processes in man. Clinically, anaerobic bacterial diseases show one or another of virtually all the cardinal features of bacterial infection, although they are not commonly communicable from man to man. Botulism stands alone since it is almost always the result of a pure intoxication that develops in the absence of an infection. At the other extreme are diseases such as Vincent's stomatitis and anaerobic streptococcal myositis in which bacterial synergism is an essential feature of the infective process.

The diagnosis of clostridial disease is not difficult and is made on clinical grounds; each of its three main forms - tetanus, gas gangrene and botulism - presenting as a characteristic clinical syndrome of systemic intoxication (Table 1).

In the last decade there has been a resurgence of interest in anaerobic bacteriology among both medical microbiologists and their clinical colleagues, due largely to an increasing recognition of the importance of the non-clostridial anaerobic bacteria as significant causes of infection in man.

The non-sporing anaerobes cause a wide variety of infections, which are most commonly initiated in the vicinity of their normal habitats (Table 2). Those most frequently encountered include anorectal and vulvo-vaginal suppurative infections; pelvic, intra-abdominal and wound sepsis following appendicectomy and gynaecological and colorectal surgery; periodontal infections; a variety of soft tissue infections; and aspiration pneumonia. Campylobacter enteritis is the most frequently encountered form of infectious diarrhoea in man.

The successful treatment of anaerobic infections in man calls for an accurate diagnosis, and this in turn depends on a close liaison between the clinician and the microbiologist. Anaerobic bacterial diseases are the subject of monographs by Finegold (1977), Smith (1977), Willis (1977); and their prevention and management by Willis <u>et al.</u> (1981).

ANTIANAEROBIC ANTIMICROBIALS

There has developed an extensive literature concerning the activity of antimicrobial agents against anaerobes. During World War II and the years immediately following, attention was confined almost entirely to the clostridia.

TABLE 1.   CLOSTRIDIA OF CLINICAL IMPORTANCE (After Willis & Phillips, 1982)

(1)   Infected wounds

Gas gangrene	Cl. perfringens type A*
	Cl. novyi type A*
	Cl. septicum
	Cl. sordellii
	Cl. histolyticum
Tetenus	Cl. tetani
Wound botulism	Cl. bolulinum
Non-pathogens**	Cl. tertium
	Cl. sporogenes
	Cl. bifermentans
	(and many others)

(2)   Enteric syndromes

Classical botulism	Cl. botulinum types A, B, E
Infant botulism	Cl. botulinum types A, B
Food poisoning	Cl. perfringens type A***
Jejunitis (Pig-bel)	Cl. perfringens type C
Enterocolitis	? Clostridium
Pseudomembranous colitis	Cl. difficile

  * Cl. perfringens type A is the commonest cause of gas gangrene
 ** The non-pathogens listed are those most commonly encountered
*** After Campylobacter enteritis, Cl. perfringens type A is the commonest cause of food poisoning

Table 2. A SUMMARY OF SOME ENDOGENOUS NON-CLOSTRIDIAL ANAEROBIC
         INFECTIONS (After Willis, 1977)

Infections of the head, neck and oropharynx
     Otitis media   )
     Sinusitis   )►Brain abscess
     Gingivitis
     Tonsillitis   )
     Cervicofacial abscess)►Bacteraemia

Pleuropulmonary infections
     Aspiration lung abscess)
     Aspiration pneumonia   )
     Metastatic lung abscess)►Thoracic empyema
     Bronchiectasis   )

Infections of the gastrointestinal tract
     Appendicitis   ) Liver abscess
     Diverticulitis   )► Subphrenic abscess
     Peritoneal soiling   ) Pelvic abscess
) Peritonitis ──► Bacteraemia

     Abdominal wound   )
     contamination   ) Wound infections
     after surgery or trauma)►Synergistic gangrene
     Perirectal abscess   ) Necrotizing fasciitis

Infections of the female genital tract
     Puerperal infection)
     Septic abortion   )►Bacteraemia
     Pelvic abscess   )
     Adnexal abscess   )►Peritonitis ──► Bacteraemia
     Endometritis ────► Pyometra

Other infections
     Gram-negative bacteraemia
     Septic arthritis and osteomyelitis
     Breast abscess, axillary abscess
     Infection of decubitus and diabetic ulcers, chronic leg
     ulcers, and ulcerating malignant lesions
     Infection of pilonidal sinus
     Paronychia
     Infected sebaceous cyst
     Human bite infections
     Addict infections
     Balanitis
     Secondary oral infections in infectious mononucleosis
     Campylobacter enteritis

Consequently, the relevant literature of this period is limited both by the small number of recognized infections and by the restricted range of drugs then available (Willis, 1969). Subsequently, in parallel with the increasing recognition of the clinical importance of non-clostridial anaerobes, interest in the spectrum of activity of antimicrobials against these organisms expanded rapidly.

Although antibiotics are properly used in the prevention and treatment of some clostridial infections, their role in these settings is usually secondary to other appropriate therapeutic or prophylactic procedures such as active immunization, passive immunization, surgery and hyperbaric oxygen therapy. Among non-clostridial anaerobic infections, on the other hand, antimicrobials are commonly of first importance both as prophylactic and therapeutic agents, and are seconded only in the event of abscess formation when surgical drainage of pus is essential.

Antimicrobial agents that act against anaerobes have been reviewed by Hamilton-Miller (1975) and Willis et al. (1981). The activity of the pricipal antibacterial agents against clinically important anaerobes is summarized in Table 3. The clinical effectiveness of some more recently introduced antimicrobials that may show impressive in vitro activity against anaerobes remains to be determined; included here are such drugs as azlocillin, cefoxatin and "augmentin" (amoxycillin/clavulanic acid). On the published evidence the claims for the clinical relevance of some of these agents to anaerobic infections seems extravagant.

CHOICE OF ANTIMICROBIAL AGENT IN TREATMENT AND PROPHYLAXIS

For many anaerobic infections there is a clear requirement for antimicrobial therapy. Absolute indications include bacteraemia, endocarditis, meningitis, pneumonia, pulmonary abscess, septic thrombophlebitis and embolic phenomena, unresolving cellulitis, acute ulcerative gingivitis and stomatitis, anaerobic streptococcal myositis, and anaerobic necretozing fasciitis and related infections. In addition, it is common practice to combine anti-biotic therapy with surgical evacuation of pus from localized infections at sites that are known to carry a special risk of bacteraemia or of thromboembolic complications; of particular importance in this respect are intraabdominal infections, pelvic sepsis associated with the female genital tract, thoracic empyema, and brain abscess. Copious pus, often associated with the formation of large abscesses, is a common finding with almost all non-clostridial anaerobic infections and the treatment of first importance in these cases is surgical drainage. It is clear in

TABLE 3 ACTIVITY OF PRINCIPAL ANTIMICROBIAL AGENTS AGAINST CLINICALLY IMPORTANT ANAEROBES

Antimicrobial	Campylobacter	Clostridium spp.	Anaerobic cocci	B. fragilis	B. melaninogenicus	Other Gram-ve bacilli
Metronidazole	+++	+++	+++	+++	+++	+++
Chloramphenicol	+++	+++	+++	+++	+++	+++
Benzylpenicillin	R	+++	+++	R	+++ or R	+++
Erythromycin	+++	+++	++	+	++	++
Clindamycin	+++	++	++	++	++	++
Carbenicillin	+++	++	+++	++	++	++
Tetracycline	+++	++	+	+	+	+
Aminoglycosides	+++	R	R	R	R	R
Vancomycin	R	+++	+++ or R	R	R	R

+++ = high and predictable activity; ++ = good but unpredictable activity; + = moderate or inconsistent activity; R = resistant

145

many instances that establishment of drainage alone may be sufficient to effect a cure, for example in drainage of dentoalveolar abscess and in surgical incision for a soft tissue abscess.

In the prophylactic setting, antimicrobials are commonly used for the prevention of tetanus and gas gangrene following accidental trauma; the prevention of postoperative gas gangrene following elective surgery about the hip and thigh, especially in elderly patients and those with obliterative arterial disease; and Cl. perfringens bacteraemia and gas gangrene of the abdominal wall following cholecystectomy. Antimicrobial prophylaxis is also widely used for the prevention of postsurgical anaerobic sepsis following colorectal surgery and appendicectomy, major gynaecological surgery (especially vaginal hysterectomy), and emergency caesarean section. Human bite wounds, and especially "closed fist" injuries carry a high risk of fulminating, destructive and even life threatening nonclostridial anaerobic infection; and for these lesions early vigorous surgical and antimicrobial prophylaxis is mandatory (Mann et al., 1977; Lancet, 1977; Goldstein et al., 1978).

Some factors that influence the choice of the antimicrobial agent include 1. the target organisms and their likely sensitivity; 2. the target tissues and the concentration of the drug attainable; 3. the susceptibility of the drug to inactivation, and its compatability with other drugs; 4. the toxicity and side effects of the drug; 5. the available routes of administration; 6. the epidemiological and ecological implications of its use; 7. the cost of the drug.

The activity of the principal antianaerobic agents against clinically important anaerobes is summarized in Table 3, and some properties of the more useful drugs in Table 4.

Target Organisms

Metronidazole, chloramphenicol and clindamycin are the most widely used drugs against anaerobes in general (Table 3); benzylpenicillin is also a valuable agent against many anaerobic bacteria, but is notably without effect on B. fragilis, campylobacter species and some strains of B. melaninogenicus (Brook et al., 1980). Metronidazole is ideally suited both to treatment and prophylaxis of anaerobic infections since it is a narrow spectrum agent that is bactericidal for the whole range of anaerobes, but with the exception of Gardnerella vaginalis, is inactive against aerobes and facultative anaerobes. Chloramphenicol, also widely and predictably active against

TABLE 4   SUMMARY OF SOME PROPERTIES OF ANTIANAEROBIC ANTIMICROBIALS

Antimicrobial Agent	Toxicity	Effect on Gut Flora	Entry into C.S.F.	Bactericidal	Route of Administration		
					Oral	Parenteral	Rectal
Metronidazole	−	−	++	++	+	+	+
Chloramphenicol	++	−	++	−	+	+	−
Penicillin	−	−	++	++	+	+	−
Erythromycin	−	+	+	−	+	+	−
Clindamycin	++	++	−	±	+	+	−
Vancomycin	++	−	−	±	+*	+	−

*Not absorbed from gastrointestinal tract

147

anaerobic bacteria, is a bacteriostatic agent that has additional broad spectrum activity against a variety of facultative anaerobes. Clindamycin is a relatively narrow spectrum bacteriostatic agent, with good activity against anaerobic organisms and most Gram-positive cocci. Erythromycin is widely regarded as the drug of choice for campylobacter infections, while oral vancomycin, which is not absorbed from the gut, has proved most effective in the treatment of Cl. difficile pseudomembranous colitis.

Target Tissues

Following administration, all of the general first line drugs - metronidazole, chloramphenicol, clindamycin and penicillin - are rapidly and widely distributed in the body, so that active levels are achieved in the tissues of the abdomen, pelvis, oropharynx, central nervous system and so on. Only clindamycin does not reach the cerebrospinal fluid.

Stability and Drug Compatability

With the exception of penicillin, which is destroyed by β-lactamase, the first line drugs are remarkably stable in vivo. The susceptibility of penicillin to β-lactamase is of therapeutic significance not only in B. fragilis and B. melaninogenicus infections, but also when mixed "passenger" organisms may protect fully penicillin-sensitive anaerobes such as Cl. tetani, Cl. perfringens and fusobacteria from the activity of the drug.

As a general guide, the scheme proposed by Mouton (1975) may be used to predict the likely effects of combining the drugs reviewed in Table 3. This system is frequently applied when blind broad spectrum therapy is provided selectively by the combined use of, say, metronidazole, gentamicin and amoxycillin. Metronidazole is exceptional among the antimicrobial agents in that it can be safely combined with virtually any other antimicrobial agent (Salem et al., 1975).

Table 5 summarizes some important incompatabilities of antianaerobic agents with other drugs.

Toxicity

Chloramphenicol is disadvantaged by its potential activity as a bone marrow depressant, clindamycin causes mild or severe diarrhoea and has been clearly incriminated in antibiotic-

TABLE 5 SOME DRUG INTERREACTIONS WITH ANTIANAEROBIC ANTIMICROBIALS

(Adapted from Stockley, 1974)

Antimicrobial Agent   Drug Interaction

METRONIDAZOLE   1. Toxic reaction with DISULFIRAM

2. Possible antabuse effect with ALCOHOL

3. Potentiates effect of ANTICOAGULANTS

CHLORAMPHENICOL 1. Reduces haemopoietic effects of IRON, FOLIC ACID, VITAMIN B$_{12}$

2. Potentiates effects of ORAL ANTICOAGULANTS

3. Potentiates action of PHENYTOIN

4. Enhances effects of ORAL HYPOGLYCAEMICS

TETRACYCLINES   1. Antibiotic effect reduced by ANTACIDS CONTAINING Al, Mg, Bi; MILK (Ca)

2. Increases nephrotoxic effects with METHOXYFLURANE

3. Antibiotic effect reduced by FERROUS SULPHATE

4. Enhances effects of ANTICOAGULANTS

5. Additive hepatotoxic effects with PHENYTOIN

6. Additive hepatotoxic effects with CHLORPROPAMIDE

7. Additive hepatotoxic effects with PHENYLBUTAZONE

CLINDAMYCIN   1. Enhances effect of NEUROMUSCULAR BLOCKERS

149

associated pseudomembranous colitis. Metronidazole is remarkably free from side effects – mild nausea, a metallic taste in the mouth and dark urine sometimes occur; long-term treatment (at least 6 weeks) may cause a reversible peripheral neuropathy.

Administration

Metronidazole, chloramphenicol, clindamycin and penicillin may all be given orally and parenterally; additionally, metronidazole may be given rectally and per colostomy as a suppository. It is clearly important that individual drugs should have alternative routes of administration that can conform to varying clinical states of the patient; for example, preoperative therapy is appropriately administered parenterally or rectally, routes that are also convenient in the unconscious, and in patients with paralytic ileus. Oral therapy is always an advantage when this is possible.

As with all antimicrobial therapy, schedules must be adequate in terms of individual dosage (to give a satisfactory peak level), dosage interval (the frequency determined by the half-life of the drug and its trough level in relation to the anticipated minimum inhibitory concentration required), and the overall duration of therapy. Anti-anaerobic antimicrobial therapy may be regarded as successful if it produces a notable clinical response within 48 hours in terms of resolution of pyrexia, tachycardia, malaise, cellulitis and pus formation. If this response is sustained, therapy may be discontinued usually in 7-10 days. The absence of such a clear and prompt response is usually due to inadequate or inappropriate antimicrobial therapy, to silent abscess formation (which requires localization and drainage before a response may be obtained or sustained), or to misdiagnosis of the nature of the infection. With certain notable exceptions e.g. brain abscess and endocarditis, prolonged antimicrobial therapy for anaerobic infections reflects diagnosis destitution or therapeutic thoughtlessness.

Epidemiological and Ecological Implications

Clindamycin therapy is commonly associated with a marked disturbance of the gut flora, and development of resistance is well known. There have been no reports of induced resistance to standard courses of metronidazole since its introduction as a trichomonaside some 18 years ago, and conventional therapy produces little detectable change in the gut flora. Since aerobic and facultatively anaerobic bacteria are inherently resistant to metronidazole, these organisms of the indigenous flora do not impose the sorts of constraints upon its use that may apply to agents of broader spectrum.

COMMENT

Because the response of the majority of anaerobes to the various first line drugs is predictable, there should rarely be any difficulty in choosing the most appropriate antimicrobial agent in particular circumstances. Because metronidazole, chloramphenicol and clindamycin are all widely active against the whole spectrum of anaerobic bacteria, these drugs may be used empirically, either when an anaerobic infection is suspected clinically or in cases of known anaerobic sepsis before the results of sensitivity tests become available. Under these circumstances, the choice of drug will be influenced by such factors as its toxicity, the required route of administration, location and severity of the infection, and concomitant aerobic infection.

For patients with severe Gram-negative sepsis, in particular those with bacteraemia, in whom antimicrobial therapy must begin before a bacteriological diagnosis is made, it may be necessary to cover the possibility of either an anaerobic or aerobic infection. In this event it is a common practice to initiate combined antimicrobial therapy, which may then be modified in the light of the bacteriological findings. One such successful regimen was clindamycin combined with gentamicin; another, which has proved equally successful but less hazardous (Lancet, 1979), is metronidazole combined with gentamicin. To either of these alternatives a penicillin may be usefully added in certain circumstances.

Although many anaerobic infections contain facultative anaerobes in addition to the predominant anaerobic flora, it is rarely necessary or desirable to use antimicrobial therapy against the facultative components. Treatment of the facultative anaerobes only, invariably fails; but antimicrobial therapy directed against the anaerobic bacteria is consistently successful. In this connection it is pertinent to recall that the mere presence of an organism in a pathological specimen does not imply an aetiological relationship to the infective process. In the same way, failure to isolate an organism does not imply its absence; many mistaken clinical diagnoses are reached as a result of misinterpretation of the bacteriological findings.

Since non-clostridial anaerobic infections of the head-and-neck and thoracic regions are commonly due to penicillin-sensitive organisms, high cure rates with benzylpenicillin may be expected in many pleuropulmonary and oropharyngeal infections. It will be realized, however, that a proportion of these infections is due to B. fragilis or to penicillin-resistant B. melaninogenicus which necessitates the use of a drug such as metronidazole. In my experience, anaerobic pulmonary infections do better when treated with metronidazole combined with amoxycillin than on metronidazole alone. In these patients meticulous physiotherapy is also an essential part of treatment. In all non-clostridial anaerobic infections that occur "below the diaphragm" it must be assumed that penicillin-resistant organisms are present.

The clinical requirements for the successful prevention and treatment of most anaerobic infections point to metronidazole as well suited to this role. It is an inexpensive, stable and readily available drug which rapidly achieves therapeutic levels in virtually all body tissues and fluids (including abscess cavities) after rectal, oral and parenteral administration. It is non-toxic and free from significant side effects, and is compatible with all other antimicrobial agents; incompatibilities with other drugs are minimal. It is bactericidal for all anaerobic microorganisms (indeed, it is the most active anti-anaerobic agent known) but is inactive against aerobes and facultative anaerobes. Coventional courses of the drug have little detectable effect on the gut flora, do not induce suprainfection and have never been known to induce resistance. The clinical and bacteriological response to metronidazole therapy is rapid, often dramatically so; patients often claim that they "feel better" within a few hours of commencing therapy; and all the clinical parameters indicate a marked improvement in 24 hours. Infected exudates are free of anaerobes in 48 hours.

I regard metronidazole as the drug of choice for all those anaerobic infections that require antimicrobial therapy.

As in many other types of bacterial infection it is helpful to control therapy by in vitro sensitivity testing. This is especially important when drugs such as erythromycin and tetracycline are in use because their activity against different strains of anaerobic bacteria are likely to be erratic. When first line drugs are used, in vitro sensitivity testing usually provides essentially confirmatory information - that the empirically selected drug, which has led to an improvement in the patient's clinical condition, is, indeed, active against the incriminated anaerobic bacteria. Such monitoring is important to guard against the possible emergence of resistant strains.

REFERENCES

Brook, I., Calhoun, L., and Yocum, P. (1980). Beta-lactamase-producing isolates of Bacteroides species from children. Antimicrob. Agents Chemother., 18, 164-166.

Finegold, S. M. (1977). Anaerobic Bacteria in Human Disease. Academic Prees, New York.

Goldstein, E. J. C., Citron, D. M., Wield, B., Blachman, U., Sutter, V. L., and Finegold, S. M. (1978). Bacteriology of human bite wounds. J. Clin. Microbiol., 8, 667-672.

Hamilton-Miller, J. M. T. (1975). Antimicrobial agents acting against anaerobes. J. Antimicrob. Chemother., 1, 273-289.

Lancet (1977). Tooth wounds and the infected fist. 1, 341-342.

Lancet (1979). Warning on antibiotic-induced colitis. 1, 1306.

Mann, R. J., Hoffeld, T. A., and Farmer, C. B. (1977). Human bites of the hand: Twenty years of experience. J. Hand Surg., 2, 97-104.

Mouton, R. P. (1975). An introduction to aspects of synergism. In The Rational Choice of Antibacterial Agents. (eds. R. P. Mouton, W. Brumfitt and J. M. T. Hamilton-Miller). Kluwer Harrap, London.

Salem, A. R., Jackson, D. D., and McFadzean, J. A. (1975). An investigation of interactions between metronidazole (Flagyl) and other antibacterial agents. J. Antimicrob. Chemother., 1, 387-391.

Smith, L. DS. (1977). Botulism. The Organism, Its Toxin, The Disease. Thomas Springfield.

Stockley, I. (1974). Drug Interactions and Their Mechanisms. Pharmaceutical Press London.

Willis, A. T. (1969). Clostridia of Wound Infection. Butterworths, London.

Willis, A. T. (1977). Anaerobic Bacteriology: Clinical and Laboratory Practice. 3rd ed. Butterworths, London.

Willis, A. T., Jones, P. H., and Reilly, S. (1981). Management of Anaerobic Infections: Prevention and Treatment. Research Studies Press, Chichester.

Willis, A. T., and Phillips, K. D. (1962). Anaerobic Bacteriology: A Bench Manual. 2nd ed. Public Health Laboratory Service Monograph Series No 3. HMSO, London.

The strategy of drug development in hypoxic cell radiosensitization and chemosensitization

I J Stratford

Radiobiology Group, Department of Physics
Institute of Cancer Research, Clifton Avenue
Sutton, Surrey SM2 5PX, UK

SUMMARY

Misonidazole (MISO, 1-(2-nitroimidazol-1-yl)-3-methoxy-propan-2-ol) is currently undergoing prospective randomized trials as a hypoxic cell sensitizer in radiotherapy. However, the neurotoxicity of this drug will limit its clinical applicability. Sensitizers with higher therapeutic ratio are therefore required. This paper outlines the experimental findings leading to the selection of MISO for clinical use. Red-ox, partition and ionization properties can affect both toxicity and radiosensitizing ability. Examples will be given where these and other properties are exploited to identify compounds likely to succeed MISO in the clinic.

It has recently been shown that MISO and other nitroaromatic compounds can <u>enhance</u> the cytotoxic action of alkylating agents <u>in vitro</u> and <u>in vivo</u>. Clinical Phase I drug combination, chemo-sensitization studies with MISO are now underway. It is apparent from experimental studies that there are nitro compounds more effective than MISO in causing this enhancement. Here, too, the importance of red-ox and partition properties will be illustrated and the more effective compounds described.

INTRODUCTION

Cells are considerably more sensitive to the lethal actions of ionizing radiation when oxygen is present during the irradiation. This action of oxygen was first demonstrated by Petry (1923). However, it was not until the detailed work of Thomlinson and Gray (1955) that it was recognized that this radiosensitizing effect of oxygen could have considerable implications in the treatment of cancer by radiotherapy. These authors postulated that hypoxic cells in solid tumours would arise as a consequence of tumour growth outstripping the vascular supply, with the hypoxic cells lying in the interface region between well-oxygenated tumour tissue and necrotic areas. Generally, hypoxic mammalian cells are around three times more radiation resistant than well aerated cells and, as a consequence, even a small percentage of hypoxic cells can profoundly influence the radiation dose required to sterilize all the tumour cells. Should hypoxic cells survive a radiation treatment they will subsequently reoxygenate and act as foci for regrowth of the tumour.

One method which may overcome this hypoxic cell problem is the use of agents which act like oxygen in increasing the radiation sensitivity of hypoxic cells. Any suitable chemical would, of necessity, have to satisfy a number of criteria before being considered for clinical use.

1) Only solid tumours contain significant numbers of hypoxic cells and any agent must only increase the radiation sensitivity of these cells, since sensitization of aerobic cells would result in increasing damage to normal tissues.

2) The compound should be relatively metabolically stable, show good uptake and tissue distribution and be able to penetrate tumours to reach the hypoxic cells likely to be lying in non-vascularized areas.

3) There should be substantial radiosensitization at doses which are non-toxic to normal tissues.

THE DEVELOPMENT OF NITROCOMPOUNDS AS RADIOSENSITIZERS

We have been guided in the search for useful chemical radio-sensitizers by our knowledge of the likely mechanism(s) by which oxygen itself can increase the radiation sensitivity of hypoxic cells. It is known from rapid-mix studies that oxygen acts in a fast free-radical process (Shenoy et al., 1975), the mechanism of which is given in Figure 1.

For this mechanism to operate it is clear that the electron affinic property of oxygen is important in increasing radiation damage. This initial suggestion (Adams and Dewey, 1963) led to the study of a large number of electron affinic compounds for their ability to sensitize hypoxic bacteria (Adams and Cooke, 1969). These agents included conjugate diketones, quinones, keto-esters, aromatic ketones and various other structures

156

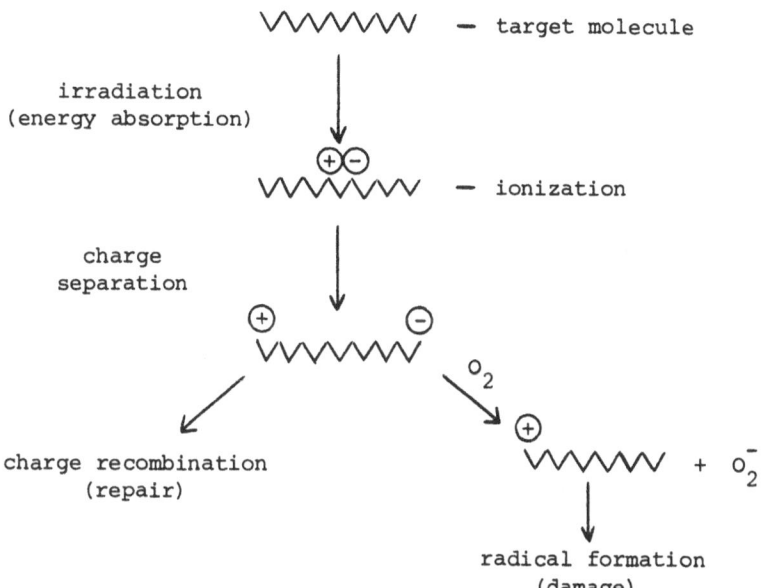

Figure 1.   The mechanism by which oxygen can increase the radiation sensitivity of cells.

containing conjugate electrophores.   In many instances, high concentrations of compounds were required to show sensitization and on very few occasions was sensitization observed in mammalian cells.   However, with the finding that p-nitroacetophenone (PNAP) provided substantial sensitization of mammalian cells in vitro at non-toxic concentrations, attention focussed on nitro compounds as potential agents for use as clinical radiosensitizers (Adams et al., 1972; Chapman et al., 1972).

In 1973 the 5-nitroimidazole, metronidazole, which was already in clinical use as an anti-trichomonal agent, was shown to give significant sensitization in vitro and in vivo (Chapman et al., 1973; Begg et al., 1973).   Subsequently, clinical evidence was presented for radiosensitization of human glioblastomas by metronidazole (Urtason et al., 1976).

Electron affinity considerations led to the suggestion that 2-nitroimidazoles should be more efficient sensitizers than their 5-nitro analogues.   This would be due to greater interaction of the nitro group in the 2- position with the π electron system of

the imidazole ring.   A number of 2-nitroimidazoles were examined
in vitro (Asquith et al., 1975) and from them misonidazole was
chosen for extensive study in vivo and eventual clinical evaluation.

At this time it is useful to relate those chemical, biological and pharmacokinetic properties of misonidazole to the criteria
we originally laid down for any compound to be useful clinically
(see Introduction).   These effects of misonidazole are detailed
as follows.
1)   Effective sensitization is seen in vitro and in vivo
using both single and multifraction radiation regimes and there
is little evidence for sensitization of aerobic cells and normal
tissues (see Fowler and Denekamp 1979 for recent review).
2)   Misonidazole is comparatively stable metabolically with
a half-life in man of around 12 hours (Flockhart et al., 1978).
In addition, the drug shows good tissue distribution and uptake
into tumours (Ash et al., 1979).
3)   Some Phase I and II clinical studies have been completed
and the drug is at present in randomized prospective trials.
However, it is apparent that NEUROTOXICITY will prevent misonidazole from being used at doses sufficiently high to give maximum
sensitization (see collected papers, Sutherland, 1982).

THE STRATEGY OF NEW SENSITIZER DEVELOPMENT

The dose limitation (12 g/m^2) that has been imposed on the
use of misonidazole has led to considerable effort in the search
for compounds that might be superior to this drug in the clinic.
There are two ways to find compounds of greater therapeutic ratio
than misonidazole.   Firstly, by maintaining the sensitizing
efficiency while reducing toxicity, thus allowing higher doses to
be given.   Secondly, by developing compounds with much greater
sensitizing efficiency.   These courses of drug development have
been followed by systematically varying different chemical parameters which would be expected to alter the biological effects of
nitroimidazoles (be it toxicity or sensitizing efficiency).

Changing Electron Affinity

The most important factor influencing sensitizing efficiency
in vitro is electron affinity.   One-electron reduction potential,
E_7^1, which is determined under equilibrium conditions by pulse
radiolysis, is a measure of electron affinity.   Figure 2A shows
that with increasing electron affinity (less negative value of E_7^1)

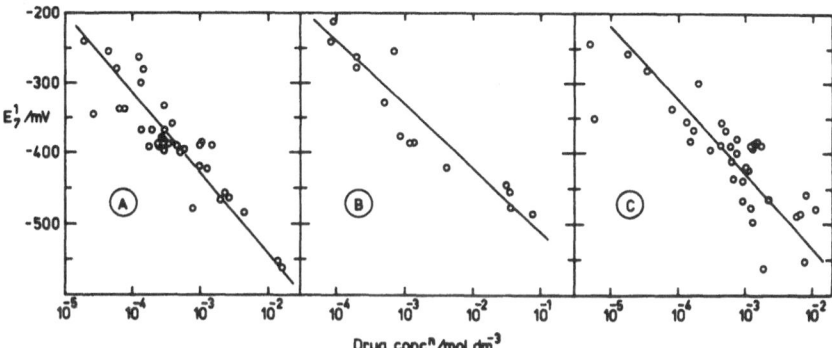

Figure 2. The effect of varying red-ox potential, E_7^1, of electron
affinic agents on their toxicity and sensitizing ability in V79
cells in vitro.   A: Sensitizing efficiency, $C_{1.6}$, the concentration of drug required to give an enhancement ratio of 1.6 (Adams,
1979a). B: Acute hypoxic toxicity at $37°C$, the concentration of
drug required to reduce surviving fraction to 10^{-2} in 5 hours
(Adams et al., 1980c). C: Chronic aerobic toxicity, the concentration required to reduce colony forming ability by 50% after
incubation in the presence of drug for 1 week (Adams et al., 1979b).

sensitizing efficiency increases, i.e. a lower concentration is
required to achieve sensitization.   This relationship appears to
hold over a wide range of sensitizing efficiencies and includes
many compounds more efficient than misonidazole.

     While the electron affinity correlation has been useful in
identifying new radiosensitizing compounds it has also shown that
toxicity increases with increasing electron affinity.   Figure
2B and 2C show the relationship between toxicity under hypoxic
conditions or chronic aerobic toxicity and red-ox potential.
Comparison of the slopes of these curves with the slope of the
sensitization curve in Figure 2A shows that the dependence upon
electron affinity for all three end-points is similar.   This in
vitro work would suggest that no improvement on misonidazole is
likely to be achieved by movement to compounds of greater electron
affinity, since toxicity will also increase.   Data from in vivo
studies support this view (Rauth and Kaufmann, 1975; Brown et al.,
1982; Sheldon, unpublished results).   These authors have examined
in tumour-bearing mice, the sensitizing and toxic effects of
nitrofurans and nitroimidazoles with greater electron affinity
than misonidazole.   All the compounds tested showed greater

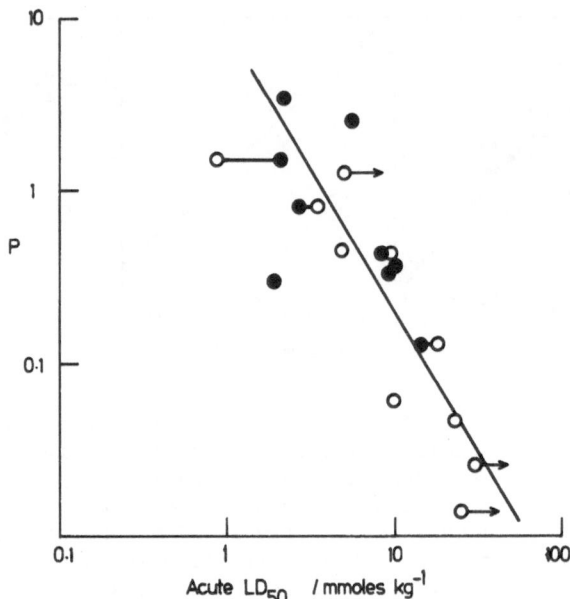

Figure 3.   The dependence of acute LD_{50} on P for a range of
2-nitroimidazoles with similar electron affinities.   Drugs were
given i.p. :   to BALB/c mice, o, (Brown and Lee, 1980);   or to
WHT mice, ●, (Sheldon, personal communication).   Bars indicate
values for the same compound in the two strains of mouse.   Arrows
indicate the maximum dose tested ($\leqslant LD_{50}$).

toxicity than misonidazole and at the concentrations tested showed
little or no sensitization.   Further, it appeared that the lack
of sensitization was probably due to the metabolic instability of
these highly electron affinic compounds.   These in vitro and
in vivo results suggest that compounds with electron affinities
similar to misonidazole are likely to be those which eventually
prove to be useful.   Consequently the development of new compounds
has proceeded by maintaining the electron affinity constant and
varying other parameters.

Changing Partition Coefficient

The octanol:water partition coefficient, P, was measured for
all the compounds illustrated in Figure 2.   These data were then

fitted to a structure activity relationship of the form

$$- \log C = b_o + b_1 E_7^1 + b_2 \log P + b_3 (\log P)^2$$

using a multiple regression analysis.   Statistical tests showed
that, for both sensitization and toxicity, the coefficients b_2
and b_3 were not significantly different from zero (Adams et al.,
1979a,b; Adams et al., 1980c).   This indicates that P, over the
range studied, had no significant effect on sensitization or
toxicity in vitro.   This lack of an involvement of P indicated
there could be considerable flexibility in drug design.   In vivo,
variations in P will cause changes in drugs' absorption, distribution, metabolism, excretion and toxicity.   A determination of
how these characteristics change as a function of P should then
allow optimization of tumour radiosensitization while sparing
toxicity to normal tissues.

The effect of changing P on the acute LD_{50} of 15 2-nitro-
imidazoles in mice is given in Figure 3.   For changes in values
of P over the range 0.014 to 3.8 there is around a 10-fold change
in toxicity with the more lipophilic compounds showing the
tendency towards greater toxicity.

In the clinic misonidazole and other nitro compounds are
neurotoxic.   In the preceding LD_{50} study some of the toxicity
appeared to be neurological.   There are a variety of methods for
testing for neurotoxicity in experimental animals and these
include morphological, behavioural and biochemical tests.   The
latter technique has been used to demonstrate the neurotoxicity
of misonidazole in rodents (Rose et al., 1980) and this method
has been adapted to study the effect of changing partition
coefficient on the neurotoxicity of nine 2-nitroimidazoles of
similar electron affinity.   These data are given in Figure 4 and
show that, for these compounds, increasing the value of P can
cause a reduction in the drug dose required to elevate
β-glucuronidase levels in the peripheral nerves of mice.   This
corresponds to the more lipophilic compounds being the more neurotoxic.

The data in Figures 3 and 4 illustrate how partition coefficient can affect the toxicity of nitroimidazoles.   In a series
of papers, Workman (1980, 1982) has shown the importance of lipophilicity in determining the pharmacokinetics of electron affinic
sensitizers and he has related changes in pharmacokinetics to
toxicity and therapeutic ratio.   In these studies compounds with
values of P from 0.014 to 30 were examined for their ability to
penetrate into the brains of experimental animals.   This was done
by taking the ratio of drug exposure to the brain, i.e. the AUC

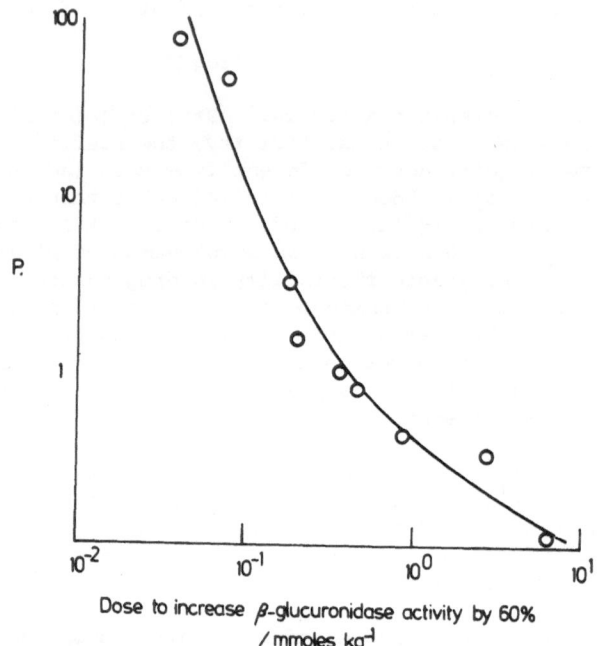

P.

Dose to increase β-glucuronidase activity by 60% / mmoles kg⁻¹

Figure 4. The dependence of neurotoxicity in C57Bl mice on the partition coefficient of a range of 2-nitroimidazoles with similar electron affinities. Drugs were given i.p. as a course of 5 daily doses. Neurotoxicity was assessed as the dose required to cause a 60% increase in β-glucuronidase activity in the distal portions of sciatic nerves of mice, 4 weeks after the cessation of drug dosing (data from Clarke et al., 1982; Adams et al., 1982).

(area under the curve of concentration x time for this tissue), compared to that for plasma. P values similar to or greater than that for misonidazole (0.43) showed ratios of around 100% indicating no tendency to concentrate in or be excluded from brain. Whereas, below 0.43 the brain to plasma ratio decreased as a function ot P, indicating that the more hydrophilic compounds were less able to penetrate the brain.

These findings are consistent with the LD_{50} and neurotoxicity results given in Figures 3 and 4 and suggest the movement to nitroimidazoles, with the same electron-affinity, but less lipophilic than misonidazole. Changing lipophilicity in this way does not alter these drugs' ability to penetrate into tumours. Brown and

Workman (1980) showed that, compared to the brain results, tumour penetration by 2-nitroimidazoles is independent of P over the range 0.026 to 3.1. Further, administration of the hydrophilic drugs by the i.v. route can result in much higher peak plasma levels than those achieved with misonidazole given either orally or i.v. Thus, in terms of therapeutic ratio, compounds of lower P will be expected to give similar levels of radiosensitization to misonidazole since similar concentrations can be achieved in tumours, but their toxicity should be considerably reduced, allowing higher doses to be given. The compound SR 2508, N-(2-hydroxyethyl)-2-(2-nitro-1-imidazolyl)-acetamide (P=0.046) has been selected from the series illustrated above and clinical studies commence shortly (Brown et al., 1981).

Changing Acid-Base Characteristics

Another method for selectively reducing tissue exposure can be by incorporating acidic or basic groups in the structure of interest. This aspect of radiosensitizer development is discussed in detail by Wardman elsewhere in these proceedings and only a brief summary is given here.

Many 2-nitroimidazoles containing heterocyclic bases in the N1 side-chain have been synthesized by Adams et al. (1980a,b) and Smithen (1980). In vitro studies showed that, generally, compounds with pKa values greater than 7.4 were more efficient sensitizers than would be predicted on electron affinity correlations. This has been attributed to increased cellular uptake of these partially ionized drugs due to concentration gradients induced by a pH differential across the plasma membrane (Wardman, 1982). Some of these compounds also show tumour to plasma ratios considerably greater than 100% and on this basis together with apparent lower neurotoxicity in vivo Ro 03-8799, 1-[3-(N-piperidino)-2-hydroxypropyl]-2-nitroimidazole, has recently entered clinical trial (Dische, personal communication).

Other Molecular Features affecting Sensitization

We have stressed earlier the importance of electron affinity in determining sensitizing efficiency. However, it is apparent from the data in Figure 2A that even within a very narrow band of red-ox potential there can be up to an order of magnitude difference in sensitizing efficiency. This has led to an examination of the properties of the compounds which show themselves to be more efficient than would be predicted from their electron affinity. One such compound was found to be 2,4-dinitro-5-aziridinyl

163

benzamide (CB 1954).   This was first synthesized as a cytotoxic agent (Khan and Ross, 1970) and was found to have both alkylating and antimetabolite properties.   CB 1954 has a similar electron affinity to misonidazole but its ability to sensitize hypoxic cells is considerably greater (Chapman et al., 1979, Stratford et al., 1981).   This extra sensitizing efficiency has been associated with the cytotoxic (presumably alkylating) activity of CB 1954 (Stratford et al., 1981).   Subsequently, other electron affinic compounds substituted with alkylating groups have been synthesized.   One of these, RSU 1069, has a similar electron affinity to misonidazole and gives enhancement ratios in vivo similar to those achieved with misonidazole but with a 10-fold lower dose (Sheldon, personal communication).   The enhanced activity of compounds of this type offer another route to the development of improved radiosensitizers.

MAKING THE MOST OF MISONIDAZOLE

Protecting against Toxicity

During the course of using misonidazole in the treatment of patients with glioblastoma, it was found that the incidence of neuropathy was significantly less in patients receiving anti-convulsants such as phenobarbitone and phenytoin or the steroid, dexamethasone (Bleehen, 1980; Wasserman et al., 1980).   It is likely that the anti-convulsants are acting by reducing the tissue exposure to misonidazole.   In experimental animals phenytoin reduces both the brain and plasma AUCs, but peak tumour levels of misonidazole are not affected (Workman, 1979).

The reason dexamethasone may protect against toxicity is uncertain.   There is some in vivo evidence to suggest that, in the presence of the steroid, the brain AUC of misonidazole is reduced in mice (Workman, 1980b).   Alternatively in vitro results suggest dexamethasone, and other anti-inflammatory agents, may protect via interference with misonidazole metabolism by a mechanism which involves inhibition of prostaglandin synthesis (Millar and Jinks, 1982).

The neurological damage caused by misonidazole in experi-mental animals has similarities with toxicities brought about by thiamine deprivation, or poisoning by acrylamide or isoniazid. Thiamine pyrophosphate, vitamin E or pyridoxin can protect against these toxicities and when given prior to and during treatment with misonidazole can result in substantial protection (Rose et al., and Brown et al., unpublished data).

Enhancing Sensitizing Efficiency

Hypoxic cells with low levels of glutathione are much more sensitive to radiation compared to normal hypoxic cells. In addition, these cells can be sensitized by misonidazole at lower concentrations than would otherwise be used (Bump et al., 1982; Stratford, 1982). There are a number of agents that can deplete cellular thiols and these include diethylmaleate (DEM), diamide and N-ethylmaleamide. Using a combination of DEM and misonidazole in vivo, greater sensitization was seen than when using either agent individually (Bump et al., 1982). This combination approach will be of value if the agents used do not have additive toxicities.

CHEMOSENSITIZATION

A property of nitrocompounds is their ability to preferentially kill hypoxic cells. The mechanism of this effect is quite different from radiosensitization and has been shown to be concentration, contact time and temperature dependent. We have noted earlier that cytotoxicity is dependent upon red-ox properties and this is indicative of the involvement of reductive processes in the mechanism. It was considered that if hypoxic tumour cells were in any way resistant to standard chemotherapy then nitro compounds may be useful in combination drug regimes (Adams and Stratford, 1981).

The use of misonidazole in combination with alkylating agents has been extensively examined both in vitro and in vivo. Typical of the data obtained is that illustrated in Figure 5 which shows the substantial enhancements that can be achieved with misonidazole and melphalan. In vivo, misonidazole itself has no apparent effect on the number of clonogenic cells per tumour but in combination with melphalan there is a marked enhancement of tumour cell kill. These results indicate that the enhanced effect using the drug combination is not due to additive toxicity but misonidazole is CHEMOSENSITIZING the action of melphalan. There is evidence to suggest potentiating effect is mediated through hypoxia since in vitro, chemosensitization is only observed when cells are given a pre-treatment with misonidazole under hypoxic conditions prior to exposure to melphalan in air (Smith et al., 1982b).

165

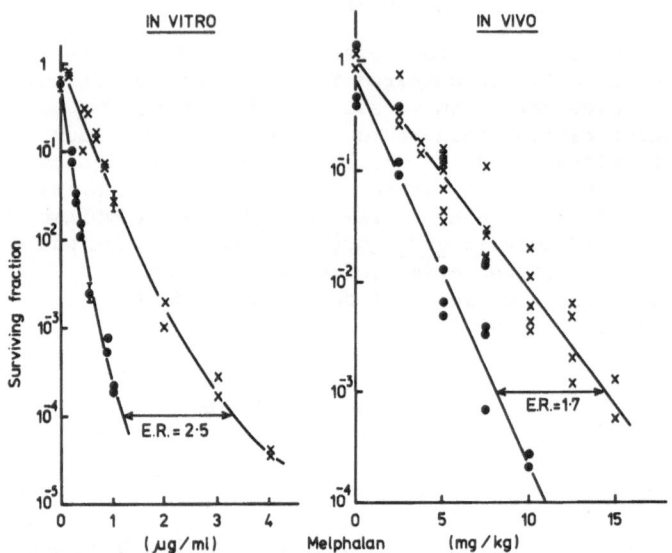

Figure 5. Chemosensitization : Misonidazole plus melphalan.
In vitro; plateau phase cells given melphalan for 1 hour at 37ºC
in air either alone, x; or after a pre-treatment with 5 mM
misonidazole for 2 hrs. under hypoxic conditions, ●; (Smith et
al., 1982b).   In vivo; mice bearing the MT tumour given
melphalan alone, x; or melphalan in combination with 2.5 mmoles/
kg misonidazole, ●; tumours were excised 24 hours after treatment
and all survival assayed in vitro. (Sheldon et al., 1982).

Misonidazole is effective in combination with most alkylating agents and the nitrosoureas (Sutherland, 1982).   However,
using these combinations there is some increase in normal tissue
damage, although it is always less than the anti-tumour effect.
Thus, there is a search for a nitro compound which will, in
combination, provide greater tumour chemosensitization than misonidazole while minimizing normal tissue damage.

This drug development program has been guided by experience
previously gained with radiosensitizers.   The effectiveness of
misonidazole has been shown to be dependent on exposure, i.e.
concentration x contact time (Smith et al., 1982b).   Further,
chemosensitization in vitro is red-ox related, with compounds of
higher electron affinity than misonidazole requiring less

exposure to cause enhancement of alkylating agent damage (Smith et al., 1982a). It was stated earlier that, <u>in vivo</u>, nitro-compounds of higher electron affinity than misonidazole show lower metabolic stability and much greater toxicity. This has led to an examination of nitro compounds with a similar red-ox potential to misonidazole but with other properties that are different.

Radiosensitization is dependent upon the concentration of drug in the tumour at the instant of irradiation, whereas chemo-sensitization depends upon the exposure to nitro compound. When partition coefficient is changed, compounds more hydrophilic than misonidazole (P < 0.43) tend to show <u>lower</u> tissue exposure, although peak levels are maintained. When given in combination with alkylating agents this results in lower activity compared to misonidazole (Workman and Twentyman, 1982). In contrast, for compounds with P values greater than 0.43 there is an increase in activity, which goes through a maximum for compounds with P values ranging from 5 to 10. This has resulted in the selection of benznidazole (P = 8.2) for use in Phase I clinical studies in combination with the nitrosourea CCNU.

CONCLUDING REMARKS

Some of the principles which have guided the development of nitro compounds for use in combination with radiation- or chemo-therapy have been outlined. In order to identify compounds superior to misonidazole it has required contributions from experts in many fields ranging from physical and synthetic organic chemistry, through pharmacology to tumour biology. This emphasizes the importance of a multidisciplinary approach being fundamental to the strategy of development of new therapeutic agents.

ACKNOWLEGEMENTS

Sincere thanks are to Christine Williamson for excellent technical assistance, Drs. Sheldon and Workman for providing unpublished results, and Sylvia Bassett and Annabel Thomas who aided in the preparation of this manuscript. Financial support from an MRC Programme Grant and an NCI Contract Grant (no. N01-CM-17485) are gratefully acknowledged.

REFERENCES

Adams, G.E., Ahmed, I., Clarke, E.D., O'Neill, P., Parrick, J., Stratford, I.J., Wallace, R.G., Wardman, P. and Watts, M.E. (1980). Structure-activity relationships in the development of hypoxic cell radiosensitizers III. Effects of basis substituents in nitroimidazole sidechains. Int. J. Radiat. Biol., 38, 613-616.

Adams, G.E., Ahmed, I., Fielden, E.M., O'Neill, P. and Stratford, I.J. (1980). The development of some nitroimidazoles as hypoxic cell radiosensitizers. Cancer Clin. Trials, 3, 37-42.

Adams, G.E., Asquith, J.C., Dewey, D.L., Foster, J.L., Michael, B.D. and Willson, R.L. (1971). Electron-affinic sensitization. II. para-Nitroacetophenone: A radiosensitizer for anoxic bacterial and mammalian cells. Int. J. Radiat. Biol., 19, 575-585 (1971).

Adams, G.E., Clarke, C., Dawson, K.B., Sheldon, P.W. and Stratford, I.J. (1982). Nitroimidazoles as hypoxic cell radiation sensitizers and cytotoxic agents. Proc. 2nd Symp.: Biological Bases and Clinical Implications of Tumour Resistance. Rome (Italy) Sept. 1980.

Adams, G.E., Clarke, E.D., Flockhart, I.R., Jacobs, R.S., Sehmi, D.S., Stratford, I.J., Wardman, P., Watts, M.E., Parrick, J., Wallace, R.G. and Smithen, C.E. (1979). Structure-activity relationships in the development of hypoxic cell radiosensitizers. I. Sensitizing efficiency. Int. J. Radiat. Biol., 35, 133-150.

Adams, G.E., Clarke, E.D., Gray, P., Jacobs, R.S., Stratford, I.J., Wardman, P., Watts, M.E., Parrick, J., Wallace, R.G. and Smithen, C.E. (1979). Structure-activity relationships in the development of hypoxic cell radiosensitizers. II. Cytotoxicity and therapeutic ratio. Int. J. Radiat. Biol., 35, 151-160.

Adams, G.E. and Cooke, M.S. (1969). Electron-affinic sensitization. I. A structural basis for chemical radiosensitizers in bacteria. Int. J. Radiat. Biol., 15, 457-471.

Adams, G.E., Dewey, D.L. (1963). Hydrated electrons and radio-biological sensitization. Bichem. Biophys. Res. Comm., 12, 473-477.

Adams, G.E. and Stratford, I.J. (1981). Hypoxia dependent radiation sensitizers and chemotherapeutic agents. In Proceedings Bristol-Myers Symp. on Molecular Actions and Targets for Cancer Chemotherapeutic Agents (eds. A.C. Sartorelli, J.R. Bertino and J.S. Lazo). Nov. 1979, pp. 401-418.

Adams, G.E., Stratford, I.J., Wallace, R.G., Wardman, P. and Watts, M.E. (1980). Toxicity of nitro compounds toward hypoxic mammalian cells: Dependence upon reduction potential. J. Natl. Cancer Inst., 64, 555-560.

Ash, D.V., Smith, M.R. and Budgen, R.D. (1979). Distribution of misonidazole in human tumours and normal tissues. Br. J. Cancer, 39, 503-509.

Asquith, J.C., Watts, M.E., Patel, K., Smithen, C.E. and Adams, G.E. (1974). Electron-affinic sensitization. V. Radiosensitization of hypoxic bacteria and mammalian cells in vitro by some nitroimidazoles and nitropyrazoles. Radiat. Res., 60, 108-118.

Begg, A.C., Sheldon, P.W. and Foster, J.L. (1973). Demonstration of radiosensitization of hypoxic cells in solid tumours by metronidazole. Br. J. Radiol., 47, 399-404.

Bleehen, N.M. (1980). The Cambridge glioma trial of misonidazole and radiation therapy with associated pharmacokinetics studies. In Radiation Sensitizers, Cancer Management 5 (ed. L.W. Brady). Masson, New York, pp. 374-380.

Brown, D.M., Yu, N.N., Brown, J.M. and Lee, W.W. (1982). In vitro and in vivo radiosensitization by 2-nitroimidazoles more electron affinic than misonidazole. Int. J. Radiat. Oncol. Biol. Phys., 8, 435-438.

Brown, J.M. and Lee, W.W. (1980). Pharmacokinetic considerations in radiosensitizer development. In Radiation Sensitizers, Cancer Management 5 (ed. L.W. Brady). Masson, New York, pp. 2-13.

Brown, J.M. and Workman, P. (1980). Partition coefficient as a guide to the development of radiosensitizers which are less toxic than misonidazole. Radiat. Res., 82, 171-190.

Brown, J.M., Yu, N.Y., Brown, D.M. and Lee, W. (1981). SR 2508: A 2-nitroimidazole amide which should be superior to misonidazole as a radiosensitizer for clinical use. Int. J. Radiat. Oncol. Biol. Phys., 7, 695-703.

Bump, E.A., Yu, N.N. and Brown, J.M. (1982). The use of drugs which deplete intracellular glutathione as radiosensitizers of hypoxic tumour cells in vivo. Int. J. Radiat. Oncol. Biol. Phys., 8, 439-442.

Chapman, J.D., Raleigh, J.A., Pedersen, J.E., Ngan, J., Shum, F.Y., Meeker, B.E. and Urtasun, R.C. (1979). Potentially three distinct roles for hypoxic cell sensitizers in the clinic. In Proc. 6th Int. Congress Radiat. Res., Tokyo, Japan (eds. S. Okada, M. Imamura, T. Terashima and H. Yamaguchi). JARR, Tokyo, pp.885-892.

Chapman, J.D., Reuvers, A.P., Borsa, J. (1973). Effectiveness of nitrofuran derivatives in sensitizing hypoxic mammalian cells to X-rays. Br. J. Radiol., 46, 623-630.

Chapman, J.D., Webb, R.G. and Borsa, J. (1971). Radiosensitization of mammalian cells by p-nitroacetopheneone. I. Characterization in asynchronous and synchronous populations. Int. J. Radiat. Biol., 19, 561-573.

Clarke, C., Dawson, K.B., Sheldon, P.W. and Ahmed, I. (1982). Neurotoxicity of radiation sensitizers in the mouse. Int. J. Radiat. Oncol. Biol. Phys., 8, 787-790.

Flockhart, I.R., Large, P., Troup, D., Malcolm, S.L. and Marten, T.R. (1978). Pharmacokinetic and metabolic studies of the hypoxic cell radiosensitizer misonidazole. Xenobiotica, 8, 97-107.

Fowler, J.R. and Denekamp, J. (1979). A review of hypoxic cell radiosensitization in experimental tumours. Pharmac. Ther., 7, 413-444.

Kahn, A.H. and Ross, W.C.J. (1969/70). Tumour growth inhibitory nitrophenylaziridines and related compounds: Structure-activity relationships. Chem. Biol. Interactions, 1, 27-47.

Millar, B.C. and Jinks, S. (1982). Protection against misonidazole induced toxicity in vitro by non-steroidal anti-inflammatory agents. Int. J. Radiat. Oncol. Biol. Phys., 8, 795-798.

Petry, E. (1923). Zur kenntnis der Bedingungen der biologischen Wirkung der Rontgenstrahlen. Biochem. Zeitschr., 135, 353-383.

Rauth, A.M. and Kaufman, K. (1975). In vivo testing of hypoxic radiosensitizers using the KHT murine tumour assayed by the lung colony technique. Br. J. Radiol., 48, 209-220.

Rose, G.P., Dewar, A.J. and Stratford, I.J. (1980). A biochemical method for assessing the neurotoxic effects of hypoxic cell radio-sensitizers: Experience with misonidazole in the rat. Br. J. Cancer, 42, 890-899.

Sheldon, P.W., Batten, E.L., Scottow, D.J. and Adams, G.E. (1982). Potentiation of melphalan activity against a murine tumour by nitroimidazoles. In press.

Shenoy, M.A., Asquith, J.C., Adams, G.E., Michael, B.D. and Watts, M.E. (1975). Time resolved effects in irradiated bacteria and mammalian cells: A rapid-mix study. Radiat. Res., 62, 498-512.

Smith, E., Lumley, C.E., Stratford, I.J. and Adams, G.E. (1982). Chemosensitization in vitro: Potentiation of melphalan toxicity by Misonidazole, Metronidazole and Nitrofurazone. Int. J. Radiat. Oncol. Biol. Phys., 8, 615-618.

Smith, E., Stratford, I.J. and Adams, G.E. (1982). The enhancing effect of misonidazole on the response to melphalan of mammalian cells in vitro. Br. J. Cancer. In press.

Smithen, C.E., Clarke, E.D., Dale, J.A., Jacobs, R.S., Wardman, P., Watts, M.E. and Woodcock, M. (1980). Novel (nitro-1-imidazolyl)-alkanolamines as potential radiosensitizers with improved therapeutic properties. In Radiation Sensitizers, Cancer Management 5, (ed. L.W. Brady). Masson, New York, pp.22-32. 32.
Stratford, U.K. (1982). Mechanisms of hypoxic cell radiosensiti-zation and the development of new compounds. Int. J. Radiat. Oncol. Biol. Phys., 8, 391-398.

Stratford, I.J., Williamson, C., Hoe, S. and Adams, G.E. (1981). Radiosensitizing and cytotoxicity studies with CB 1954 (2,4-dinitro-5-aziridinylbenzamide). Radiat. Res., 88, 502-509.

Sutherland, R.L. (1982). Conference on Chemical Modification: Radiation and Cytotoxic Drugs. Int. J. Radiat. Oncol. Biol. Phys., 8, 323-815.

Thomlinson, R.H., Gray, L.H.(1955)Histological structure of some human lung cancers and the possible implication for radiotherapy. Br. J. Cancer, 9, 539-549.

Urtasun, R.C., Band, P., Chapman, J.D., Feldstein, M.L., Mielke, B. and Fryer, C. (1976). Radiation and high dose metronidazole (Flagyl) in supratentorial glioblastomas. New Engl. N. Med., 293, 1364.

Wardman, P. (1982). Molecular structure and biological activity of hypoxic cell radiosensitizers and hypoxia specific cytotoxins. In Advanced Topics on Radiosensitizers of Hypoxic Cells (eds. A. Breccia, C. Rimondi and G.E. Adams). NATO Advanced Study Institutes Series A43. Plenum, New York, pp.49-76.

Wasserman, T.H., Phillips, T.L., van Raalte, G.V., Urtasun, R.C., Partington, J., Kozio, A., Schwade, J.G., Ganji, D., Strong, J.M. (1980). The neurotoxicity of misonidazole: Potential modifying role of phenytoin sodium and dexamethasone. Br. J. Radiol., 53, 172-173.

Workman, P. (1979). Effects of pre-treatment w phenobarbitone and phenytoin on the pharmacokinetics and toxicity of misonidazole in mice. Br. J. Cancer, 40, 335-345.

Workman, P. (1980). Pharmacokinetics of hypoxic cell radio-sensitizers: A review. Cancer Clin. Trials, 3, 237-251.

Workman, P. (1980). Drug interactions with misonidazole: Effects of dexamethasone and its derivatives on the pharmacokinetics and toxicity of misonidazole in mice. Biochem. Pharmac., 29, 2769-2776.

Workman, P. (1982). Lipophilicity and the pharmacokinetics of nitroimidazoles. In Advanced Topics on Radiosensitizers of Hypoxic Cells (eds. A. Breccia, C. Rimondi and G.E. Adams). NATO Advanced Study Institutes Series A43. Plenum, New York, pp. 143-163.

Workman, P. and Twentyman, P.R. (1982). Enhancement by electron-affinic agents of the therapeutic effects of cytotoxic agents against the KHT tumour: Structure-activity relationships. Int. J. Radiat. Oncol. Biol. Phys., 8, 623-627.

Quantitative structure-activity relationships (QSARs): Principle and practice

P Wardman

Cancer Research Campaign, Gray Laboratory
Mount Vernon Hospital, Northwood
Middlesex HA6 2RN, UK

INTRODUCTION

The desire to relate differences in the biological effects of xenobiotic compounds to particular chemical properties can be stimulated by one or other of two interrelated, but nonetheless distinct goals. On the one hand, the aim may be to collate data on the chemical structures and biological activities of existing compounds, with a view to identifying new compounds with improved therapeutic properties - the end being more important than the means. On the other hand, the desire to introduce new drugs may be less important than an interest in the mechanisms of action of existing compounds - the end being a better understanding of the properties of the target and its biological host.

Hansch and Fujita (1964) suggested "...the hypothesis that... biological effects resulting from structural changes can be correlated by means of regression analyses with two parameters, σ [an electronic term] and π [a lipid:water partition term], seems well worth further study." Since then, numerous quantitative structure-activity relationships (QSARs) between chemical properties and biological activity have been published. This brief article is written not for the practitioner of QSAR - for whom Martin (1981) has provided a recent perspective - but for those who have a practical use of the approaches developed by QSAR specialists but are, in effect, "frightened off" by the language, nomenclature and statistical skills which appear to be necessary.

The purpose of this article is not, therefore, to preach to the converted. Rather, it aims to fill the gap between no knowledge of the subject, and the numerous, detailed expositions of the principles and techniques which have been published. In recent years the

173

author has himself crossed this gap and it is hoped that a distill-
ation of this experience may be useful to those who stand on the
edge.

RELATIONSHIPS BETWEEN DRUG STRUCTURE AND BIOLOGICAL ACTIVITY

Quantifying the Biological Response

Relationships between structure and activity will usually take
the general form:

$$\text{biological activity} = \text{function(s) of chemical properties} \quad (1)$$

The chemical concepts of rate and equilibrium - both practically
defined in terms of concentration - are central to the description
of appropriate chemical properties to be used in equation (1), and
in practice there are sound reasons why the method of biological
testing should enable drug activity or potency to be expressed in
terms of the dose or concentration required to achieve a constant,
defined biological response. This requires multiple measurements
of response and dose, although transformation of limited data of
response at a fixed dose is sometimes possible using logit trans-
formations or other assumptions (e.g. Martin, 1978; Chu, 1980). In
all the examples given below, the molar concentration C required for
a fixed response has been interpolated from multiple measurements.

Free Energy as the Basis for Differences in Activity

Drug activity depends upon a series of individual steps -
dissolution, absorption, distribution, drug-receptor binding (or
reaction with the target), metabolism, excretion, etc. - most of
which are individually amenable to treatment by established concepts
based upon free energy, i.e. upon chemical equilibria. Free energy
is an additive concept, and variations in overall activity (i.e. in
overall chemical properties) are separable into the effects of free-
energy changes associated with different properties. We can write:

$$\text{biological activity} = \text{function(s) of electronic + partition +}$$
$$\text{steric + ionization +...terms} \quad (2)$$

The method now commonly known as Hansch Analysis (e.g. Hansch, 1971;
Gould, 1972; Martin, 1978) requires numerical values for the individual terms in equation (2), and uses multivariate analysis to assess
the relative importance of each chemical property upon the overall
biological response.

It is important to recognise that: (i) different algebraic forms may be appropriate to describe the dependence of drug activity upon different properties - linear, quadratic, logarithmic, bilinear etc.; (ii) the inclusion of terms relating drug activity to any individual molecular property may reflect contributions from several phenomena to drug activity. Thus hydrophobicity, as characterized by lipid:water partition terms, may influence not only drug transport and phase equilibria, but also, e.g. drug/receptor binding when the target is in a hydrophobic environment; (iii) interrelationships between chemical properties may complicate the analysis and even lead to false conclusions.

Free and Wilson (1964) made no assumptions as to the relative importance of individual physico-chemical _properties_ to the overall biological activity, but used multiple regression analysis with dummy variables to determine the effect of a particular _group_ at any one position in a molecule or base structure. Pattern-recognition methods also offer an alternative approach (Martin, 1978; Chu, 1980). However, most QSARs rely upon multiple linear regression to examine statements of the form of equation (2), i.e. Hansch Analysis, and this method is illustrated below. We outline first the estimation of the chemical parameters required in the equation and then turn to the problem of the mathematical steps required in the analysis.

MEASUREMENT AND PREDICTION OF CHEMICAL PARAMETERS WHICH CONTROL THE BIOLOGICAL RESPONSE

Electronic Parameters

Many QSARs investigate the behaviour of series of analogues in which one particular substituent is varied. In such circumstances it is convenient to use the Hammett substituent constant, σ (or a variant) as an electronic parameter:

$$\log K_X - \log K_H = \rho\, \sigma_X \qquad (3)$$

where σ_X reflects the shift in position of an appropriate equilibrium caused by the replacement of H in the molecule by a substituent X (Hammett, 1970). Whilst Hansch (1971) noted that "Attempts to extend the Hammett equation to biochemical systems have been most disappointing" and interest in hydrophobic (partition) effects still dominates QSAR research, in the author's Laboratory investigations of the use of nitroaromatic compounds as hypoxic cell sensitizers for radiotherapy and as specific hypoxic cell toxins revealed that electronic properties dominated the biological response (see below). Since a variety of (nitro)aromatic structures were of interest - and subsequent extension to non-nitro electron-affinic compounds was anticipated - the substituent constant approach was of limited value as it would require a knowledge of the effect of varying X in quite different systems and the "normalisation" constants ρ were unknown. We therefore measured the electron affinity of the molecule as a whole, in aqueous solution at pH 7, as the one-electron reduction potential (E) determined under thermodynamically reversible conditions.

Since adding one electron to nitroaromatic compounds yields a free radical of limited lifetime in aqueous solution, the technique of pulse radiolysis was used to estimate the positions of redox equilibria in a few microseconds after radical formation (see e.g. Wardman, 1978). Such measurements were especially relevant to these applications because the compounds were thought to radiosensitize by fast, free-radical reactions involving the transfer of a single electron (e.g. Adams and Cooke, 1969; Simic and Powers, 1974; Wardman, 1977; Willson, 1981). Further, the nitro free radical was demonstrated to be the obligate intermediate in the nitroreduction of metronidazole, nitrofurantoin, etc. by microsomal preparations (Mason, 1979), and one-electron transfer from the nitro free radical to oxygen is thought to be the basis for the selective toxicity of such compounds to anaerobes and to hypoxic cells (see Mason, 1979; Wardman and Clarke, 1976a). The value of the pulse radiolysis method in measuring the energetics of reduction to a free radical, a process thought to be involved in controlling the biological response, illustrates the potential of sophisticated yet conceptually simple approaches in the choice of chemical parameters with which to compare the biological response.

Once measurements of a suitable chemical property have been made for selected representatives of a series of compounds, the Hammett equation (3) may be used to predict the values for unknown members of the same series in many instances. Figure 1 illustrates that the reduction potential, E of 5-substituted 1-methyl-2-nitro-imidazoles and of 4-substituted nitrobenzenes varies linearly with the Hammett σ_p^- value of the substituent obtained from the literature (Hansch and Leo, 1979) and originally derived from the pK_a's of benzenoid compounds applied to equation (3).

Partition Parameters

Fujita et al. (1964) defined a new substituent constant, π, to describe the effects of a substituent X on the lipophilicity or octanol:water partition constant, P of a molecule:

$$\log P_X - \log P_H = \pi_X \tag{4}$$

an equation used in the same manner as the Hammett relationship.

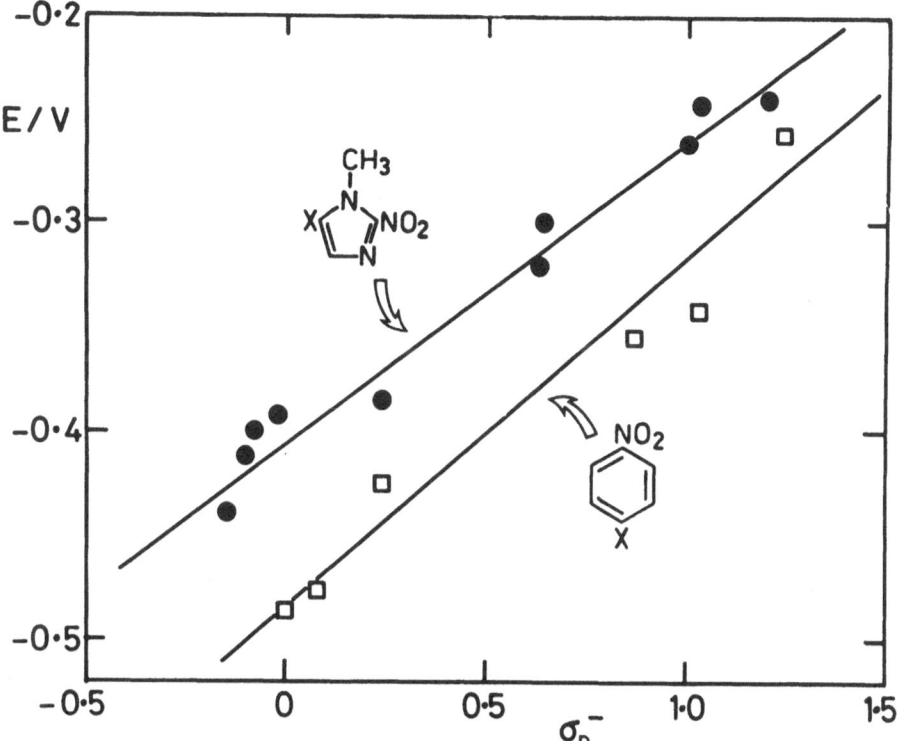

Figure 1. Dependence of measurements of the one-electron
reduction potential, E of nitro compounds in water at pH 7 upon the
Hammett σ_p values of the substituent (see Wardman (1982) for references).

As described above in connexion with estimation of parameters for
electronic effects, when series of molecules with a common "base"
structure are included in the same study, only limited experimental
measurements of partition coefficients (e.g. octanol:water) will be
necessary. Literature values of π (Hansch and Leo, 1979) for the
substituents of interest will generally enable good estimates of
the partition coefficients to be interpolated from plots of log P
vs. π_X as illustrated in Figure 2. (Part of these data were shown
in a preliminary report (Wardman et al., 1978; Fig. 1) which
gives details of the substituents X used, and more extensive data
of the same type were summarized by Wardman (1982).)

    More recently, a variant of the Hansch π approach - use of
fragmental constants (f) to calculate log P - has attracted attention (e.g. Rekker, 1977; Hansch and Leo, 1979). In the series of

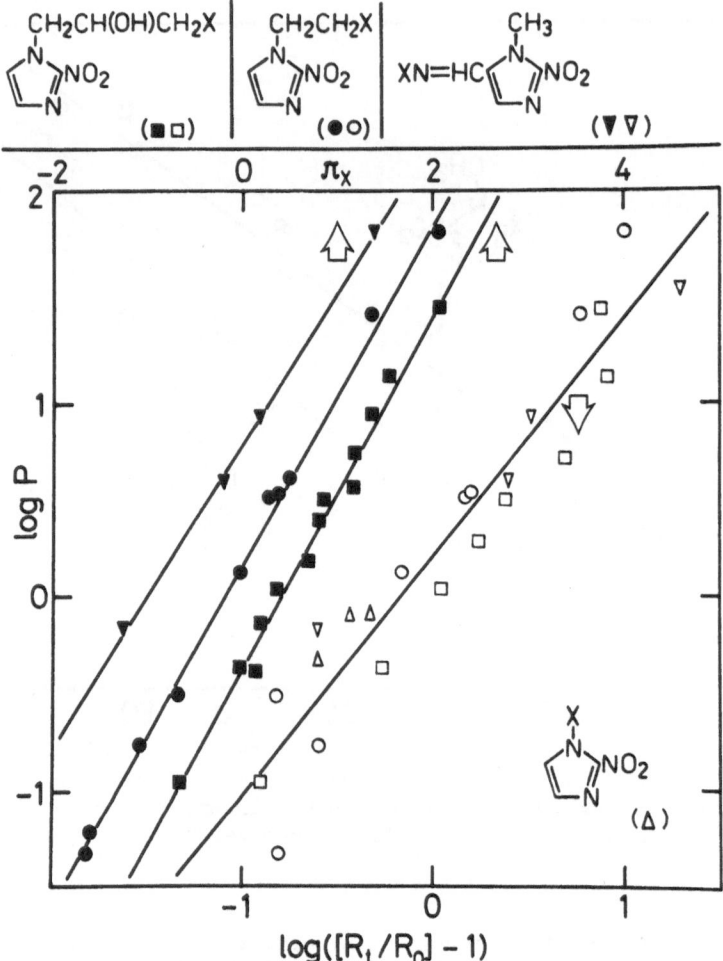

Figure 2. Dependence of measurements of the octanol:water partition coefficients, P of some nitroimidazoles upon the Hansch parameter, π_x (solid symbols, upper scale) or upon a chromatographic retention parameter (open symbols, lower scale, see text).

compounds shown in Figure 2, the more extensive π values gave at least as good predictions of log P, once a few baseline measurements were made, in spite of the fact that π values are generally derived from substituted benzenes whereas in these examples the group X terminates a 2- or 3-atom aliphatic chain. Figure 2 also compares measured values of log P with a chromatographic retention parameter. High performance liquid chromatography on a Spherisorb ODS 10 μm column using methanol:water (40:60) gave values for the retention time R_t from which an appropriate parameter could be calculated, allowing for the system retention R_o (McCall, 1975). These unpublished measurements from the author's Laboratory (kindly supplied by Mr. R. A'Court and Dr. M.R.L. Stratford) illustrate that reasonable estimates of log P can be made using readily-available columns. There is no doubt that the uncertainties associated with this method of interpolating estimates of log P from measurements with a few compounds can be much reduced from those illustrated in this preliminary investigation, e.g. by more complete silylation (McCall, 1975) or by the use of a column coated with octanol (Unger et al., 1978).

Steric Parameters

Adding steric parameters to a proposed QSAR already incorporating a lipophilicity (partition) term or function immediately introduces a new problem. Unless great care is taken with the choice of substituents in the design of congener sets, collinearity between variables may lead to false conclusions. As a simple example, increasing the size of an alkyl substituent will usually lead to an increase in lipophilicity. If partition effects are important in controlling the biological response, an apparent influence of steric parameters may be concluded because the two properties are related in the set of compounds studied. This problem has been discussed in detail by Hansch and Leo (1979), who also compared the various measures of steric effects useful for incorporating in QSARs.

Prototropic Effects

Since electronic effects are often quantified via the Hammett equation based upon prototropic equilibria - acid dissociation or base protonation, in some QSARs involving acids or bases, pK_a may be used as a variable. Whether this variable then reflects the importance of prototropic effects or merely the influence of groups which are electron-donating or withdrawing and which influence another reaction centre in addition to an acidic or basic function may not be easy to determine. Martin (1978) has discussed in detail several possible ways in which QSARs involving acids or bases may be developed. In the author's Laboratory the importance of prototropic equilibria in controlling pH-induced concentration gradients across cell membranes has been demonstrated in some recent studies which will be outlined later.

Other molecular properties which could be used as variables in equations of the form of (2), and much more detailed discussion of the factors outlined above, can be found in e.g. Martin (1978), Hansch and Leo (1979) and Yalkowsky et al. (1980).

THE TECHNIQUE OF MULTIVARIATE ANALYSIS

The text by Draper and Smith (1966) cannot be recommended too highly; other useful texts are Snedecor and Cochran (1967) and Overall and Klett (1972), and Martin (1978).

Least-Squares Fit to a Straight Line

Most physical scientists are familiar with the use of least-squares methods to fit the "best" straight line through n sets of data points, $(x_1,y_1),(x_2,y_2)...(x_n,y_n)$. The simplest approach to QSAR using the Hansch approach would be to examine the correlation between biological activity expressed in concentration terms and each possible chemical variable in turn. Thus a possible influence of redox properties might be sought for by fitting the data to an equation of the form:

$$\log(1/C) = -\log C = b_0 + b_1 E \qquad (5)$$

where C is the concentration required for a defined response, E the reduction potential and b_0 and b_1 are the estimates of the intercept and slope of the least-squares fit to the data. The first chapter of Draper and Smith (1966) explains the procedures for an unbiased test of the significance of regression using an F-test or by testing the null hypothesis that b_1 is equal to zero (no relationship between log C and E) using a two-sided t-test. The result of such tests is the probability that the relationship observed (if any) could have arose purely by chance.

Additional Variables: Multiple Linear Regression

It is when we need to examine the effects of two or more independent (chemical) variables upon a single (biological) response that many baulk at the computational or statistical skills apparently involved. This is a great pity, since relatively cheap microcomputers can now be purchased with a Matrix ROM (Read-Only Memory) which performs all the necessary manipulations using simple BASIC commands no longer than this paragraph. With a little homework on matrix algebra, once complex multivariate analyses can be approached with confidence.

Whilst Chapter 2 of Draper and Smith (1966), presenting linear regression in matrix form, may appear difficult to some at first sight, the matrix solution to the problem is so useful - and now so easy to execute - that its advantages completely outweigh any initial difficulties met.

If we have n data sets of a dependent (biological response) variable Y_k each with m corresponding (chemical) parameters $(X_{1,k}, X_{2,k}...X_{m,k})$ then the solution we seek is:

$$\hat{Y} = b_0 + b_1 X_1 + b_2 X_2 + ... b_m X_m \qquad (6)$$

where $\hat{Y}$ is the predicted value of the biological response Y for a given set of $(X_1, X_2...X_m)$, i.e. chemical properties. We wish to determine the individual values of the coefficients $(b_0, b_1, b_2...b_m)$, the variance associated with each value so we can ascertain if it is statistically non-zero, and the extent to which the variation in the overall (biological) response is explained by each individual chemical parameter.

In matrix terms we begin by defining a vector $\underline{Y}$ to be the n (row) by 1 (column) array listing the values $(Y_1, Y_2...Y_n)$. (In the text here we use underlining to denote a matrix or vector - an array in the BASIC program illustrated below.) The matrix $\underline{X}$ is a n (row) x (m+1) (column) array listing the values:

$$
\begin{array}{ccccc}
1 & X_{1,1} & X_{2,1} & \cdots & X_{m,1} \\
\vdots & \vdots & \vdots & & \vdots \\
1 & X_{1,n} & X_{2,n} & \cdots & X_{m,n}
\end{array}
$$

Lines 10 to 30 in the example below dimensions the arrays and fills them from the data file stored on disc or cassette. One can easily extend the instructions to include only selected compounds or a defined set of chemical properties.

```
...10 REM MAT A = Y, MAT B = X
   20 DIM A(n,1), B(n,m+1)
   30 REM SUBROUTINE TO FILL ARRAYS FROM DATA FILE ETC.
   40 MAT C = TRN(B):MAT D = C*B:MAT E = INV(D)
   50 MAT F = C*A:MAT G = E*F:MAT PRINT G
```

The solution $(b_0, b_1...b_m)$ is a vector denoted as $\underline{b}$ which is an array of (m+1) rows and one column given by:

$$\underline{b} = (\underline{X}'\underline{X})^{-1}\underline{X}'\underline{Y} \qquad (7)$$

where $\underline{X}'$ is the transpose of matrix $\underline{X}$ (obtained in line 40 as MAT C using the TRN coding), $\underline{X}'\underline{X}$ is the product MAT D of matrix $\underline{X}$ with its transpose, and $(\underline{X}'\underline{X})$ is then inverted using the INV coding giving MAT E. MAT F is the product $\underline{X}'\underline{Y}$ and when multiplied by MAT E yields the desired result, printed out as a single column of m rows listing the values of $b_0, b_1...b_m$ using the MAT PRINT instruction in line 50.

The built-in BASIC commands to multiply, transpose, invert,

redimension and print the various matrices and vectors reduce the computational skills required to a minimum, only the rules for multiplication of matrices requiring a little care (MAT D = C*B is correct but MAT D = B*C is not, in the example here).

The mean square s^2 (the estimate of σ^2) is then easily calculated with few additional instructions as:

$$s^2 = (\underline{Y}'\underline{Y} - \underline{b}'\underline{X}'\underline{Y}) / (n - m - 1) \tag{8}$$

and the estimates of the variance (= the square of the estimated standard error) of the individual coefficients $b_0, b_1 \ldots b_m$ obtained as the diagonal elements of the matrix:

$$\underline{V}(\underline{b}) = (\underline{X}'\underline{X})^{-1} s^2 \tag{9}$$

These estimated standard errors (est.s.e., the square roots of the variances) can then be used in two-sided t-tests to ascertain whether the null hypotheses: $b_0, b_1 \ldots b_m = 0$ can be rejected at any chosen level of probability.

We evaluate in each case the t-statistic:

$$t = b_i / (\text{est.s.e. } b_i) \tag{10}$$

and compare $|t|$ with $t(n-m-1, 1-\tfrac{1}{2}\alpha)$ from a t-table. We have $(n-m-1)$ degrees of freedom and the test is at the $100(1-\alpha)$ % probability level. As a rule of thumb, unless the number of data sets n less the number of (chemical) variables m is less than 10, the t-statistic calculated from equation (10) has to exceed ca. 2.3 if the hypothesis that $b_i = 0$ is to be rejected at the 95 % confidence level.

Another statistic often used in QSAR is the (multiple) correlation coefficient R or its square, given by:

$$R^2 = (\underline{b}'\underline{X}'\underline{Y} - n\,\bar{Y}^2) / (\underline{Y}'\underline{Y} - n\,\bar{Y}^2) \tag{11}$$

where $\bar{Y}$ is the mean value of Y. Generally, if a (chemical) variable is to be useful in predicting biological response in a QSAR, then its incorporation in the equation should increase R. We note, however, that the use of R as a measure of "goodness of fit" has been criticized (Davis and Pryor, 1976) and a sequential F-test is easily incorporated in a program involving stepwise addition of each chosen variable (see e.g. Martin, 1978).

It is hoped that this brief description of the matrix approach to multiple regression illustrates the simplicity of the programming required if a Matrix ROM is available to perform the matrix algebra under BASIC commands, which could also test for collinearity between

the chemical parameters of interest using e.g. a squared correlation
matrix (Hansch and Leo, 1979). The same approach can be used with
non-linear functions, e.g. by treating log P and $(log P)^2$ as two
independent variables; Berntsson (1980) discussed the previously-
neglected problem of covariability between such linear and squared
terms.

TWO EXAMPLES WHERE A SINGLE CHEMICAL PROPERTY
DOMINATES THE BIOLOGICAL RESPONSE

Radiosensitization of Mammalian Cells by Nitroaromatic Compounds

Raleigh et al. (1973) studied the radiosensitization (increased
cell killing) caused by a series of substituted nitrobenzenes with
hypoxic Chinese hamster V79 cells in vitro. They showed that the
biological response at a fixed concentration of nitro compound
increased with the electron-withdrawing power of the substituent,
as characterized by its Hammett σ constant.

In extending these studies to nitroimidazoles and other aromatic
systems of potentially greater clinical usefulness, Adams et al.
(1976) utilized the pulse radiolysis method to establish relative
one-electron reduction potentials as previously described by Meisel
and Neta (1975) for nitro compounds (Wardman and Clarke, 1976b).
Figure 3 illustrates how useful these measurements were in enabling

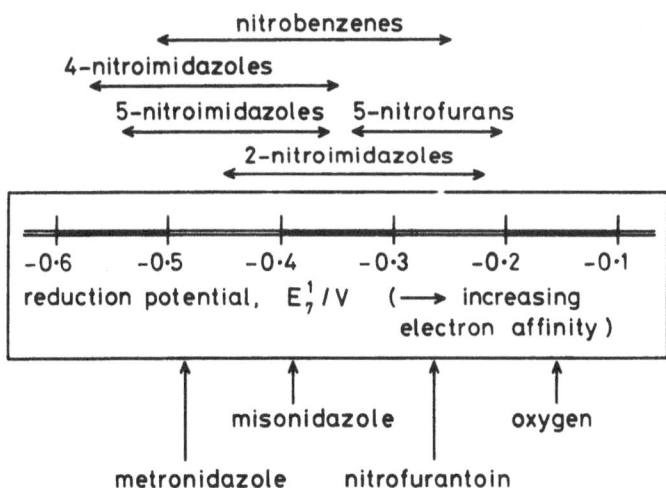

Figure 3. Scale of electron affinity (one-electron reduction
potential vs. NHE in water at pH 7) for nitroaromatic compounds.

different structural types to be related to a common scale; we have already demonstrated (Figure 1) how Hammett substituent constants can be used to estimate reduction potentials once measurements have been made for representative members of a series.

In extensions of this use of reduction potential in correlating redox properties with biological response, Adams et al. (1979a,b; 1980) fitted their data to a QSAR of the form:

$$- \log C = b_0 + b_1 E \tag{12}$$

where C was the molar concentration in the extracellular medium required to achieve a constant biological response. These 3 papers described how the one equation could successfully describe measurements not only of the radiosensitization efficiency of nitroaromatic compounds, but also measurements of both chronic aerobic and hypoxic cytotoxicity of the compounds towards the same cells in vitro.

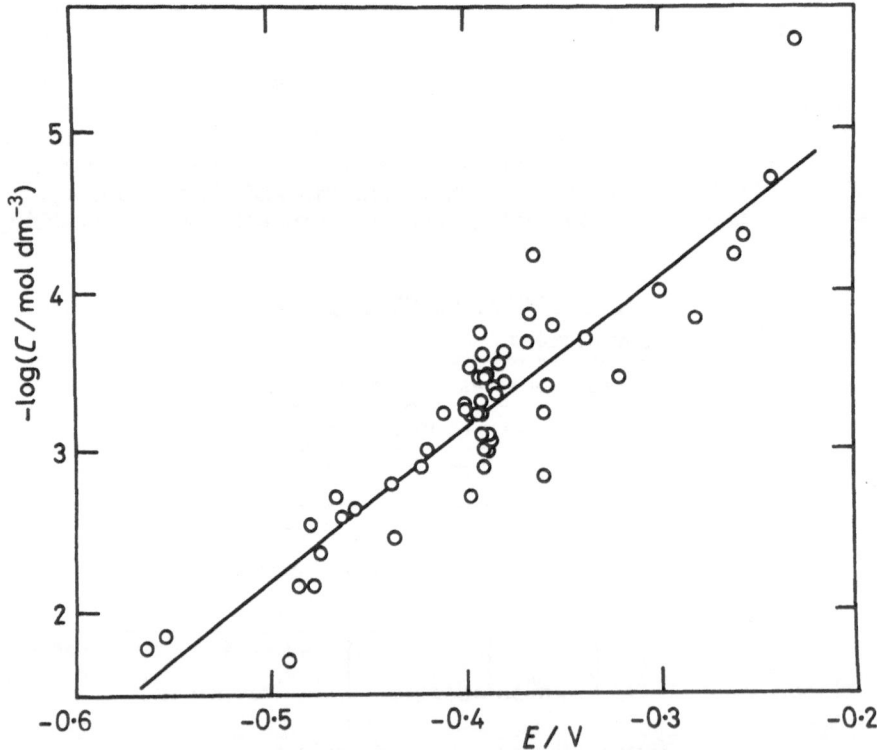

Figure 4. Relationship between the concentration C required to achieve a constant radiosensitization response and the reduction potential E of nitroaromatic compounds (see Wardman, 1982).

Interestingly, the slopes b_1 of all three QSARs were similar:
8.21 ± 0.57, 8.40 ± 0.91, and 10.1 ± 1.0 for E expressed in
volts. Wardman (1981) drew attention to the mechanistic implications
of the quantitatively similar redox dependences observed for these
and several other biological properties of nitroaromatic compounds.

Including further data accumulated by the same group, Wardman
(1982) fitted radiosensitization data for 56 such compounds to
equation (12), yielding:

$$- \log C = (6.96 \pm 0.22) + (9.54 \pm 0.56) \, E/V \qquad (13)$$

with R = 0.918 and s = 0.272. These data are plotted in Figure 4;
the scatter around the least-squares fitted line arises in part from
the concentration-dependence of the biological response and the
uncertainty in measurements of the latter. These factors should
always be taken into account when analysing the results from QSARs.

Searching for possible effects of lipophilicity by fitting the
data to the multivariate equation:

$$- \log C = b_0 + b_1 E + b_2 \log P + b_3 (\log P)^2 \qquad (14)$$

yielded coefficients: $b_1 = 9.45 \pm 0.57$, $b_2 = 0.098 \pm 0.077$, and
$b_3 = -0.043 \pm 0.072$. As noted earlier, for significance at the
95 % confidence level the standard errors shown with each coefficient
need to be at least two-fold smaller than the coefficients, in order
that the null hypothesis: $b_i = 0$ may be rejected. Hence the data
do not demonstrate an influence of partition terms - which is not
the same as saying that the data demonstrate no influence of partition! (R was fractionally increased using equation (14) to 0.921
and s remained constant at 0.272.)

The compounds included in the analyses above covered quite a
wide range of octanol:water partition coefficients, P (from about
0.1 to 100). However, when extremely polar compounds were studied
(P < 0.05), a reduced response was noted which was thought to arise
from reduced uptake into the cell. We shall return to this problem
of extracellular/intracellular concentration gradients later.

Activity of Nitroimidazoles towards Trichomonas foetus

In complete contrast to the example above, partition properties
were shown by Butler et al. (1967) to dominate the efficiency of a
series of 5-nitroimidazoles with varying 2-alkyl substituents in
treating mice infected with Trichomonas foetus. The effects on the
reduction potential E of varying the 2-substituent R in the series
of compounds shown in Figure 5 would be very small; they can be

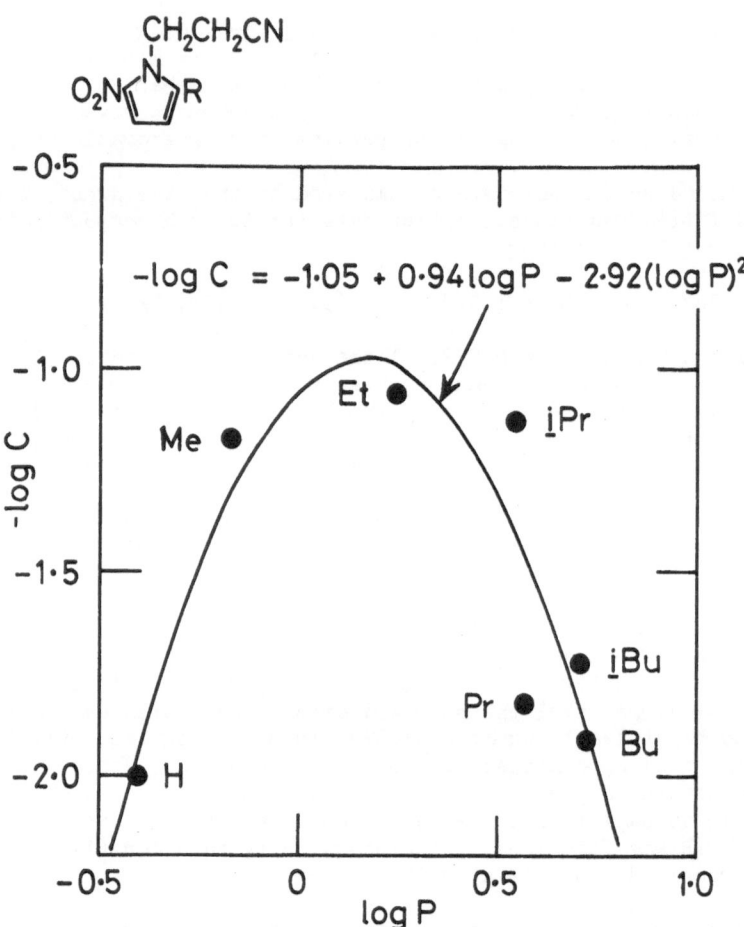

Figure 5. Activity of some 5-nitroimidazoles towards T. foetus when administered to mice. C is the dose (mg/kg) required for a 50 % cure rate and P the octanol:water partition coefficient. (Data from Butler at al., 1967).

estimated to a first approximation from the upper line in Figure 1, which describes the redox properties of a related series. The Hammett σ_p of R varies from 0 for H to ca. -0.16 for the higher alkyls, so that E will vary by no more than 0.023 V. The line drawn through the data in Figure 5 is the parabola of the form:

$$- \log C = b_0 + b_1 \log P + b_2 (\log P)^2 \qquad (15)$$

yielding R = 0.860.

Most discussions of the effects of ionization of acids (HA) or protonation of bases (B) upon biological activity are centred around the concept of the conjugates (HA/A⁻ or BH⁺/B) reacting with a receptor with differing efficiencies. Martin (1978) discusses this approach in some detail. In some other studies, effects of ionization equilibria in reality describe the importance of the electronic term in the QSAR, since the interrelationship between ionization and redox properties is the basis for the classical Hammett equation.

Figure 6 illustrates a dramatic effect of ionization phenomena observed in the author's Laboratory, with two radiosensitizers. The two compounds differ only in the circled groups; the methyl substituent in the imidazolyl ring of 8-nitrocaffeine is replaced by H in 8-nitrotheophylline. The concentrations required to achieve a radiosensitization factor of e.g. 1.2 differ by ca. 5 orders of magnitude. Measurements of the one-electron reduction potential, E show a decrease of 0.29 V results from this substitution of CH_3 by H, and from the experience with neutral compounds described by equation (13), one can calculate that a decrease of about 600-fold in radiosensitization efficiency would be expected - much less than

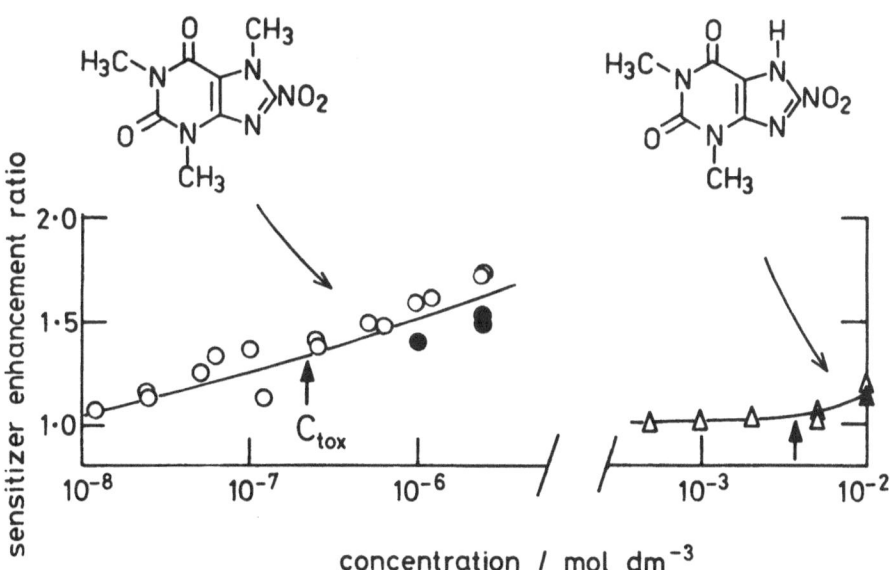

Figure 6. Radiosensitization of hypoxic mammalian cells in vitro by 8-nitrocaffeine (left) and 8-nitrotheophylline (right). Data from Wardman et al. (1980).

was observed.

The answer to this problem lies in the prototropic properties of 8-nitrotheophylline (right) not available when alkylated (left); the N-H bond ionizes with $pK_a = 2.3$, so that only ca. 0.001 % of 8-nitrotheophylline is undissociated at pH 7.4 and the anion A^- is extremely polar, slowing down intracellular uptake. In addition, a pH-induced concentration gradient will be generated which excludes the compound (including both HA and A^-) from the cytoplasm relative to the extracellular medium.

If the external membrane of the cell is permeable to the uncharged species HA or B but not to the charged conjugates A^- or BH^+, then if the interior of the cell is at a different pH (pH_i) relative to the extracellular fluid (pH_e), then it is readily shown (see e.g. Wardman (1982)) that there will be an intracellular:extracellular concentration gradient with ratio $C_i:C_e$ given by:

$$C_i/C_e = (1 + 10^{pH_i-pK}) / (1 + 10^{pH_e-pK}) \qquad \text{(acid)} \qquad (16)$$

$$C_i/C_e = (1 + 10^{pK-pH_i}) / (1 + 10^{pK-pH_e}) \qquad \text{(base)} \qquad (17)$$

where K is the equilibrium constant ($= 10^{-pK_a}$) for the dissociation of the acids HA or BH^+.

If the pK_a of the acid/base equilibria are sufficiently displaced from the pH's of the system - in this case say one unit away from 7.4 - then equations (16) and (17) approximate to:

$$C_i/C_e \simeq 10^{pH_i-pH_e} \qquad \text{(acid)} \qquad (18)$$

$$C_i/C_e \simeq 10^{pH_e-pH_i} \qquad \text{(base)} \qquad (19)$$

There is considerable evidence (Roos and Boron, 1981) that the intracellular pH in mammalian cells in culture is in the region of 7.1, i.e. ca. 0.3 units below the extracellular pH in the assay system used in the author's Laboratory. Hence there should be a ca. 2-fold concentration of e.g. weak bases with $pK_a \geqslant 8$ inside the cell, as calculated from equation (17) or its approximate form (19).

Wardman (1982), noting that 25 out of 27 nitroimidazoles substituted with basic side chains ($pK_a > 7.4$) were more efficient radiosensitizers than equation (13) predicted - based upon the extracellular concentrations C_{nom} nominally assumed to equal the intracellular concentrations only for neutral compounds of moderate lipophilicity - therefore suggested that pH-induced concentration gradients should be allowed for by combining equation (12) with (16) or (17) as appropriate:

$$-\log(C_{nom}[C_i/C_e]) = (6.81 \pm 0.20) + (9.15 \pm 0.51)\ E/V \qquad (20)$$

which then described the behaviour of 90 compounds, neutral, acids and bases, with R = 0.887 and s = 0.291. Measurements of intracellular concentrations and the variation of radiosensitization with extracellular pH confirmed the validity of this approach (Clarke et al., 1982; Watts and Jones, 1981).

CONCLUSION

In attempting to bridge the gap between the novice and the specialist in QSAR, we have seen how an appropriate selection of physico-chemical properties and an appreciation of the chemical properties of the biological target can be useful in correlating variations in biological properties with chemical parameters. Many QSARs attempt to link activity in only a single series of compounds, so that the use of substituent constants alone - e.g. π and σ - are frequently successful. With the use of modern microcomputers, only a few lines of BASIC instruction can be sufficient to make detailed statistical analyses of the relative contribution of individual chemical properties to the overall biological response.

ACKNOWLEDGEMENTS

This work is supported by the Cancer Research Campaign. I am grateful to all my colleagues who have contributed to the work which is referred to in this paper.

REFERENCES

Adams, G.E. and Cooke, M.S. (1969). Electron-affinic sensitization. I. A structural basis for chemical radiosensitizers in bacteria. Int. J. Radiat. Biol., 15, 457-471.

Adams, G.E., Flockhart, I.R., Smithen, C.E., Stratford, I.J., Wardman, P. and Watts, M.E. (1976). Electron-affinic sensitization. VII. A correlation between structures, one-reduction potentials, and efficiencies of nitroimidazoles as hypoxic cell radiosensitizers. Radiat. Res., 67, 9-20.

Adams, G.E., Clarke, E.D., Flockhart, I.R., Jacobs, R.S., Sehmi, D.S. Stratford, I.R., Wardman, P. and Watts, M.E. (1979a). Structure activity relationships in the development of hypoxic cell radiosensitizers. I. Sensitization efficiency. Int. J. Radiat. Biol., 35, 133-150.

Adams, G.E., Clarke, E.D., Gray, P., Jacobs, R.S., Stratford, I.J., Wardman, P., Watts, M.E., Parrick, J., Wallace, R.G. and C.E.

Smithen. (1979b). Structure-activity relationships in the development of hypoxic cell radiosensitizers. II. Cytotoxicity and therapeutic ratio. Int. J. Radiat. Biol., 35, 151-160.

Adams, G.E., Stratford, I.J., Wallace, R.G., Wardman, P. and Watts, M.E. (1980). Toxicity of nitro compounds towards hypoxic mammalian cells in vitro: dependence on reduction potential. J. Natl. Cancer Inst., 64, 555-560.

Berntsson, P. (1980). The use of non-correlated log P and (log P)^2 values in quantitative structure activity relationships. Acta Pharm. Suec., 17, 199-208.

Butler, K., Howes, H.L., Lynch, J.E. and Pirie, D.K. (1967). Nitroimidazole derivatives. Relationship between structure and antitrichomonal activity. J. Med. Chem., 10, 891-897.

Chu, C.C. (1980). The quantitative analysis of structure-activity relationships. In Burger's Medicinal Chemistry, Fourth Edition, Part 1, The Basis of Medicinal Chemistry. (ed. M. E. Wolff). Wiley, New York.

Clarke, E.D., Dennis, M.F., Jones, N.R., Minchinton, A.I., Stratford, M.R.L., Wardman, P. and Watts, M.E. (1982). The importance of pH-induced concentration gradients in the use of nitroimidazole radiosensitizers with basic and acidic substituents. Br. J. Radiol., in the press.

Davis, Jr., W.H. and Pryor, W.A. (1976). Measures of goodness of fit in linear free energy relationships. J. Chem. Educ., 53, 285-6.

Draper, N.R. and Smith, H. (1966). Applied Regression Analysis. Wiley, New York.

Free, S.M. and Wilson, J.W. (1964). A mathematical contribution to structure-activity studies. J. Med. Chem., 13, 1184-1189.

Fujita, T., Iwasa, J. and Hansch, C. (1964). A new substituent constant, π, derived from partition coefficients. J. Amer. Chem. Soc., 86, 5175-5180.

Gould, R.F. (ed.) (1972) Biological Correlations - The Hansch Approach. (Adv. Chem. Ser., 114). Amer. Chem. Soc., Washington.

Hammett, L.P. (1970). Physical Organic Chemistry. Reaction Rates, Equilibria, and Mechanisms. 2nd edn. McGraw-Hill Kogakusha, Tokyo.

Hansch, C. (1971). Quantitative structure-activity relationships in drug design. In Drug Design, vol. 1 (ed. E.J. Ariëns). Academic Press, New York.

Hansch, C. and Fujita, T. (1964). ρ-σ-π Analysis. A method for the correlation of biological activity and biological structure. J. Amer. Chem. Soc., 86, 1616-1626.

Hansch, C. and Leo, A. (1979). Substituent Constants for Correlation Analysis in Chemistry and Biology. Wiley, New York.

Martin, Y.C. (1978). Quantitative Drug Design. A Critical Introduction. Dekker, New York.

Martin, Y.C. (1981). A practitioner's perspective of the role of quantitative structure-activity analysis in medicinal chemistry. J. Med. Chem., 24, 229-237.

Mason, R.P. (1979). Free radical metabolites of foreign compounds and their toxicological significance. Rev. Biochem. Toxicol., 1, 151-200.

McCall, J.M. (1975). Liquid-liquid partition coefficients by high-pressure liquid chromatography. J. Med. Chem., 18, 549-552.

Meisel, D. and Neta, P. (1975). One-electron redox potentials of nitro compounds and radiosensitizers. Correlation with spin densities of their radical anions. J. Amer. Chem. Soc., 97, 5198-5203.

Overall, J. E. and Klett, C.J. (1972). Applied Multivariate Analysis. McGraw-Hill, New York.

Raleigh, J.A., Chapman, J.D., Borsa, J., Kremers, W. and Reuvers, A.P. (1973). Radiosensitization of mammalian cells by p-nitro-acetophenone. III. Effectiveness of nitrobenzene analogues. Int. J. Radiat. Biol., 23, 377-387.

Rekker, R.F. (1977). The Hydrophobic Fragmental Constant. Elsevier, Amsterdam.

Roos, A. and Boron, W.F. (1981). Intracellular pH. Physiol. Revs., 61, 296-434.

Simic, M. and Powers, E.L. (1974). Correlation of the efficiencies of some radiation sensitizers and their redox potentials. Int. J. Radiat. Biol., 26, 87-90.

Snedecor, G.W. and Cochran, W.G. (1967). Statistical Methods, 6th edn. Iowa State University Press, Ames.

Unger, S.H., Cook, J.R., and Hollenberg, J.S. (1978). Simple proce-dure for determining octanol-aqueous partition, distribution, and ionization coefficients by reversed-phase high-pressure liquid chromatography. J. Pharm. Sci., 67, 1364-1366.

Wardman, P. (1977). The use of nitroaromatic compounds as hypoxic cell radiosensitizers. Current Topics Radiat. Res. Q., 11, 347-398.

Wardman, P. (1978). Application of pulse radiolysis methods to study the reactions and structure of biomolecules. Rep. Prog. Phys., 41, 259-302.

Wardman, P. (1981). Oxygen-like radiosensitizing drugs: importance of free-energy relationships. In Oxygen and Oxy-Radicals in Chemistry and Biology. (eds. M.A.J. Rodgers and E.L.Powers). Academic Press, New York.

Wardman, P. and Clarke, E.D. (1976a). Oxygen inhibition of nitro-reductase: electron transfer from nitro radical-anions to oxygen. Biochem. Biophys. Res. Commun., 69, 942-949.

Wardman, P. and Clarke, E.D. (1976b). One-electron reduction pot-entials of substituted nitroimidazoles measured by pulse rad-iolysis. J. Chem. Soc. Faraday Trans. I, 72, 1377-1390.

Wardman, P., Clarke, E.D., Flockhart, I.R. and Wallace, R.G. (1978). The rationale for the development of improved hypoxic cell radiosensitizers. Br. J. Cancer, 37 (Suppl.3), 1-5.

Wardman, P., Clarke, E.D., Jacobs, R.S., Minchinton, A.I., Stratford, M.R.L., Watts, M.E., Woodcock, M., Moazzam, M., Parrick, J.,

Wallace, R.G. and Smithen, C.E. (1980). Development of hypoxic cell radiosensitizers. The second and third generations. In Radiation Sensitizers. Their Use in the Clinical Management of Cancer. (ed. L.W. Brady). Masson, New York.

Wardman, P. (1982). Molecular structure and biological activity of hypoxic cell radiosensitizers and hypoxic-specific cytotoxins. In Advanced Topics in Hypoxic Cell Radiosensitization. (eds. G.E. Adams, A. Breccia, and C. Rimondi). Plenum Press, New York.

Watts, M.E. and Jones, N.R. (1981). Radiosensitization of hypoxic mammalian cells by nitroimidazoles with acidic and basic substituents: the effects of extracellular pH. Radiat. Res., $\underline{87}$, 479.

Willson, R.L. (1981). Oxygen-like radiosensitizers: mechanisms of action. In Oxygen and Oxy-Radicals in Chemistry and Biology. (eds. M.A.J. Rodgers and E.L. Powers). Academic Press, New York.

Yalkowsky, S.H., Sinkula, A.A., and Valvani, S.C. (1980). (eds.) Physical Chemical Properties of Drugs. Dekker, New York.

Three-dimensional aspects of molecules in drug design

J P Tollenaere

Department of Theoretical Medicinal Chemistry
Janssen Pharmaceutica, B-2340 Beerse, Belgium

INTRODUCTION

Although "drug design" in the literal sense of the word is
overly optimistic, todays' drug-designer can search for trends in
biological data as a function of the structural features of the
molecules exhibiting a given biological activity with the
ultimate objective of a more rational approach to the planning of
new compounds (Cramer, 1980; Martin, 1981). Once a relationship
between biological activity and structure is found, one may
extrapolate the data by synthesizing and testing a new compound
with increased amounts of hopefully activity increasing
structural features. As it is not possible to change only one
property of a molecule, introduction of a single additional
structural element will induce an appreciable change in many
other properties of the molecule. An example will make this
clear. When a NO_2-group is introduced in the para-position of
say phenoxyacetic acid, one will observe a change in the
lipophilicity, the pKa-value, the charge distribution over the
molecule, the dipole moment and the molar volume of the new
compound. If the NO_2-group is introduced at the ortho-position
of the phenyl ring, not only the above physical quantities but
the conformation of the molecule as well will be changed. In
other words, a medicinal chemist will be faced with a highly
complex data set of dimensionality n.

Mathematical techniques are available, however, enabling to
disentangle and to extract useful SAR's (Structure-Activity
Relationships). The most favoured quantititative SAR (QSAR)
method is that pioneered by Hansch (Hansch and Fujita, 1964) and
subsequently shown to be a powerful method to analyze biological
data in terms of lipophilic, electronic and steric effects

(Hansch and Leo, 1979). The Hansch method has been successfully used in the rationalization of the uncoupling activity of substituted salicylanilides, benzimidazoles and phenols (Tollenaere, 1973) and in a comparative study of the SAR of substituted phenols as uncouplers of oxidative phosphorylation in rat liver and Ascaris suum muscle mitochondria (Tollenaere et al., 1976).

From the theoretical point of view, a serious limitation of the QSAR approach lies in the description suitable for QSAR work of the three-dimensional aspects of molecules. Until recently, no extrathermodynamic terms were available which effectively described the conformational degree of freedom and the variation of conformation induced by substitution. In fact, Hopfinger (1980), Battershell et al. (1981) and Hopfinger (1982) pioneered QSAR studies on dihydrofolate reductase inhibition by Baker triazines, and substituted quinazolines and a QSAR study for a set of 1-(X-phenyl)3,3-dialkyltriazenes for which mutagenic potency was reported, based on molecular shape analysis (MSA). The basis of MSA is to determine the common steric overlap volume between pairs of molecules as a function of their conformation and relative intermolecular geometry. As MSA requires the spatial atomic coordinates of the molecule, immediately the question arises as to how the conformation of a molecule will be determined.

The aim of this contribution is to show how the various techniques of conformational and the subsequent description of molecular structure may lead to a better understanding of the factors involved when drugs interact with a putative receptor.

CONFORMATIONAL ANALYSIS

Conformational analysis in drug design is not an end in itself but rather the beginning and the basis for answering the question concerning the biologically relevant conformation, or the preferred conformation at the receptor site. In practice, three methods are available to determine the conformation of molecules in the three aggregation states. These are X-ray crystallographic analysis for the solid state, quantum chemical or empirical calculations for the isolated state and to a lesser extent nuclear magnetic resonance (NMR) analysis for the liquid or dissolved state (Tollenaere, 1981).

X-Ray Diffraction Analysis

Single-crystal X-ray diffraction analysis is the method of

194

choice for determining the three-dimensional structure of a molecule (Tollenaere et al., 1979). Although a very detailed description of the molecular geometry is obtained with the modern equipment of today, X-ray diffraction analysis usually yields only one conformation a molecule can adopt and tells us nothing about others possibly equienergetic or secondary conformations and their relative stabilities. Inspection and analysis of the molecular packing arrangements in the unit cell may yield some valuable information regarding the sites of inter- and intramolecular hydrogen bonds.

NMR Analysis

In principle, NMR analysis yields the conformation of a substance in solution. Due to the molecular complexity of many drug molecules, the interpretation of an NMR spectrum is seldom straight forward and in many cases leads to a partial solution of the conformational characteristics of the solute molecule.

Quantum Chemical and Empirical Calculations

Quantum chemical calculations yield in principle the whole conformational domain of a molecule in the isolated state, the relative stabilities or energy of each of the conformers, the orbital energy levels (e.g. Highest Occupied Molecular Orbital and Lowest Empty Molecular Orbital), the charge distribution and any other quantity derivable from the wave functions. Owing to the computational costs of quantum chemical calculations the exploration of the conformational domain is usually restricted to a few rotational degrees of freedom. But even so, theoretical conformational analysis may uncover a number of alternative conformations which are equienergetic or nearly so with observed conformations. At dramatically reduced costs one may perform empirical or molecular mechanics calculations which merely yield the purely conformational aspects of a molecule. Although it is outside the scope of this article to discuss the merits and the shortcomings of the various theoretical approaches to conformational analysis it is safe to state that the quantum chemical approach especially those of ab initio quality is to be preferred over the empirical calculations unless they are extremely well parameterized. The choice between the empirical and non- or semiempirical schemes will be chiefly dictated by the size of the molecule and the type of answer wanted.

The "Fourth" Aggregation State of Drug Molecules

　　None of the three techniques available for the determination
of the conformation of a molecule in the three aggregation states
tell us something about the biologically relevant conformation.
In principle, the three techniques may yield us an inventory of
all the conformations of the conformational domain of a
molecule. There is no a priori reason, however, to assume that
any of these three is a good approximation of what may be called
the medicinal chemist's "fourth" aggregation state or that
particular inter- and intramolecular arrangement of drug
molecules in the biophase or at the site of the receptor. It may
be argued that the conformation of a drug molecule in the
"fourth" aggregation state could be appreciably different from
any of the experimentally observed conformations. For instance
it may be severely questioned whether the isolated state with the
implicit assumption of a dielectric constant $\varepsilon = 1$ of the
surrounding medium bears any resemblance to the state of a
molecule residing in an environment of lipids and proteins.
Conformational results based on NMR experiments conducted in
aqueous or chloroform solutions are equally suspect if water or
chloroform are considered as model compounds mimicking the
surrounding environment of the drug molecule.

　　Although in many cases X-ray and NMR analysis point towards
the same predominant conformer, examples are known where both
experimental techniques indicate different conformers.
Discrepancies also exist between the results of the theoretical
approach and the two experimental methods. It is well
established that in many cases these discrepancies can be
explained when the theoretical method takes into account the
prevailing experimental environmental conditions of the liquid or
solid state. Thus the possible discrepancies between the results
of the theoretical approach and the two experimental methods are
not necessarily a reflection of the unreliability of the former
(Tollenaere et al., 1980).

　　In conclusion, it should be emphasized that conformational
analysis carried out by a concerted experimental and theoretical
approach permits the determination of the conformation of a
molecule in three different environments. Subsequent correlation
studies are necessary to investigate whether the experimentally
and/or theoretically derived conformations are of biological
relevance.

　　One recent example should suffice to illustrate the power of
the combined approach of X-ray diffraction and NMR techniques in
conformational analysis. Fig. 1 shows the classical
2-dimensional structure of ivermectin a potent broad-spectrum

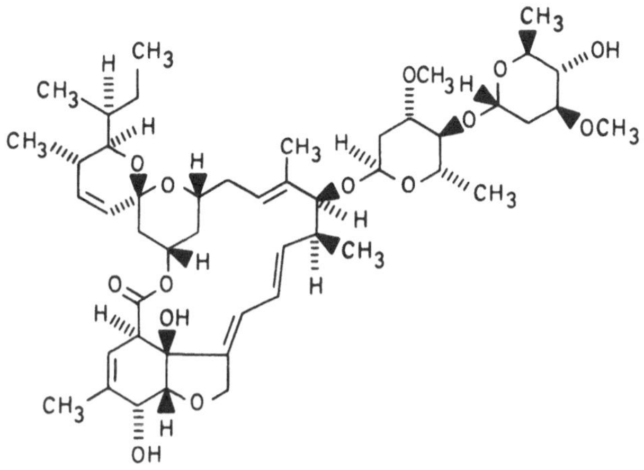

Fig. 1. Two-dimensional structure of ivermectin.

anthelmintic with ectoparasitic activity (Chabala et al., 1980; Albers-Schonberg et al., 1981). Detailed ^{1}H NMR analysis showed the conformation of the skeleton of ivermectin in solution to agree very well with the conformation observed in the solid state. Fig. 2 shows ivermectin with the correct absolute configuration.

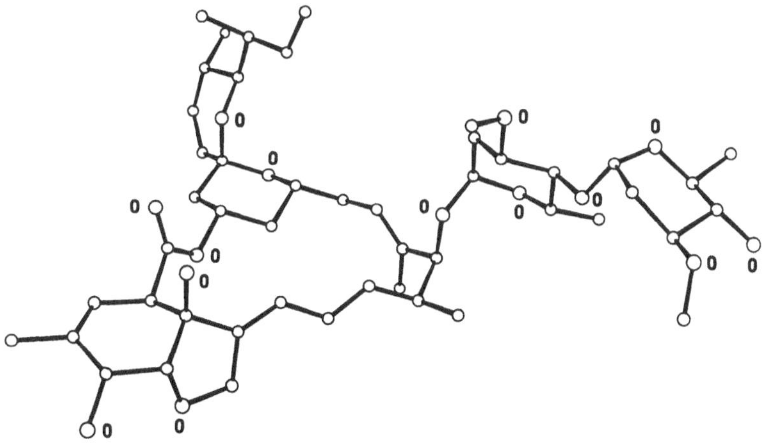

Fig. 2. Perspective drawing of ivermectin based on X-ray crystallographic data. The hydrogen atoms are omitted for clarity.

NON—BONDED INTERACTIONS

The forces governing the interactions between drug molecules and receptor site moieties are those generally occurring between various types of molecules. The only difference between drug-receptor interactions and interactions of ordinary organic chemicals is one of degree only: the resultant energy of the former is a complex function of many more energy contributions than that of the classical organic chemical reaction. In this paragraph a brief discussion will be presented of the various interaction energies involved.

Electrostatic Interactions

The monopole-monopole interaction energy of two charges Q_1 and Q_2 separated by a distance r immersed in a medium of dielectric constant ε is given by

$$E = \frac{1}{\varepsilon} \frac{332\ Q_1\ Q_2}{r} \quad \text{Kcal/mole} \tag{1}$$

where 332 is a conversion factor which expresses E in Kcal/mole when r has the dimension Å. As eq. 1 shows an inverse power relationship with respect to r, monopole-monopole, or charge—charge interactions are rather long range interactions.

A cation and an anion separated by 5 Å in vacuum ($\varepsilon = 1$) would have an interaction energy of -66.3 Kcal/mole.

Ion-Dipole Interactions

The ion-dipole interaction shown in Fig. 3 is governed by the relationship represented by eq. 2 where $\mu = Q_d l$ is the dipole moment expressed in Debye units

$$E = \frac{69.1}{\varepsilon} \frac{Q\ \mu\ \cos\theta}{r^2} \quad \text{Kcal/mole} \tag{2}$$

$$l << r$$

The ion-dipole interaction energy is of the order of -1.95 Kcal/mole for $Q = -1$, $\theta = 45°$, $\mu = 1$ D, $\varepsilon = 1$ and $r = 5$ Å.

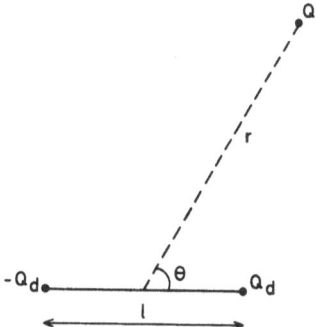

Fig. 3. Interaction between an ion with charge Q and a dipole
$\mu = Q_d l$ separated by a distance r.

Dipole-Dipole Interactions

The potential energy of two dipoles in a fixed mutual
orientation not only depends on the distance between them but
also on their relative orientations (see Fig. 4). The
interaction energy is given by

$$E = -\frac{14.4}{\varepsilon} \frac{\mu_a \mu_b}{r^3} (2 \cos \theta_1 \cos \theta_2 - \sin \theta_1 \sin \theta_2) \text{ Kcal/mole} \quad (3)$$

$$l << r$$

The energy of two dipoles $\mu = 1$ D in vacuum at a distance of
5 Å in an orientation for maximal interaction (i.e. $\theta_1 = \theta_2 = 0°$)
is of the order of -0.23 Kcal/mole.

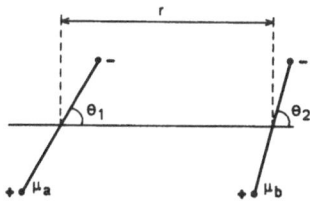

Fig. 4. Interaction of dipoles μ_a and μ_b separated by
distance r.

Hydrogen Bond

Although the hydrogen bond is still a much debated subject it suffices to note that the hydrogen bond is an intermediate range intermolecular interaction between an electron deficient hydrogen atom and electronegative elements such as F, Cl, O and N. The hydrogen bond energy is of the order of 2-10 Kcal/mole (Kollman and Allen, 1972). Due to its probably electrostatic nature the hydrogen bond energy will vary with changes of pH and the ionic strength of the surrounding medium. The quantitative, albeit empirical form of the hydrogen bond potential may be represented by eq. 4 (McGuire et al., 1972)

$$E_{HB} = \frac{-A'}{r^{10}} + \frac{B'}{r^{12}} \tag{4}$$

where the first term represents the attractive part and the second the repulsive part of the potential and where r is the distance H...Y in XH...Y.

Ion-Induced Dipole Interactions

All molecules in an electric field created by a charge Q become polarized resulting in a dipole whose moment is dependent on the field strength and the properties of the molecule. It can be shown that the energy of this type of interaction is given by

$$E = \frac{-166}{\varepsilon^2} \frac{\alpha_0 Q^2}{r^4} \quad Kcal/mole \tag{5}$$

where α is the polarizability of the molecule.

The interaction energy of a water molecule ($\alpha_0 = 1.444$) in the field of a monovalent cation or anion at a distance of 5 Å in vacuum is of the order of -0.38 Kcal/mole.

Dipole-Induced Dipole Interactions

In the same fashion as a dipole can be polarized by a monopole, a dipole will be polarized by another dipole. The maximal energy of interaction between two identical dipoles μ separated by a distance r is given by

$$E = \frac{-14.4}{\varepsilon^2} \frac{2\alpha_0 \mu^2}{r^6} \quad (Kcal/mole) \tag{6}$$

200

Two water molecules (μ = 1.83 D) 5 Å apart would involve a
dipole-induced dipole interaction energy of -0.009 Kcal/mole.

Dispersion, London or Van der Waals Interactions

Neutral non-polar molecules attract one another up to certain
distances. Upon closer intermolecular distances smaller than the
sum of the Van der Waals radii of the two approaching atoms
strong repulsion is observed. A popular form modeling the
attraction and the repulsion upon too close contact is given by a
Lennard-Jones potential of general form

$$E = -\frac{A}{r^6} + \frac{B}{r^{12}} \tag{7}$$

where A and B are empirical constants for the attractive and the
repulsive part respectively. Fig. 5 represents a typical Van der
Waals interaction curve showing the variation of E as a function
of the separation between two oxygen atoms. The minimum energy is
seen to be E = -0.345 Kcal/mole at the equilibrium distance r =
2.82 Å.

In summary, non-bonded interactions are numerous. The
relatively largest contribution to the total interaction energy
arises from monopole-monopole or electrostatic interactions.
Furthermore, it is seen that all interactions are of general form
$1/r^n$ where n = 1, 2, 3, 4, 6, 10, and 12. The interactions do
not only depend on an inverse distance relationship but do also
depend on mutual orientation angles. It follows that the
energetics of the approach of a drug molecule towards a receptor
site and eventually the final docking of the drug is an extremely
complex function of the mutual geometry of the forming complex of

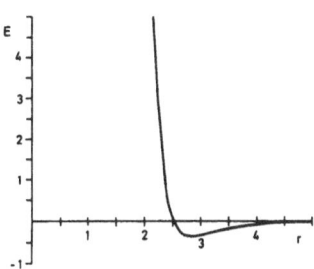

Fig. 5. Van der Waals interaction E as a function of the
separation r between two oxygen atoms. The constants A and B of
eq. 7 (see text) have been taken from Stuper et al., 1979.

the drug and receptor. The more so if it is assumed that both
drug and receptor may mutually adapt their conformations during
the approach phase.

DRUG-RECEPTOR INTERACTION

In order to gain a better understanding of drug-induced
conformational changes in a receptor, it is extremely
illustrative to discuss in some detail a recent study by Aubry et
al. (1981). These authors observed that the model tripeptide
t-Bu-CO-L-Pro-Me-D-Ala-NHMe crystallizes in both the anhydrous
(A) and hydrated forms (A.H_2O).

Let us assume for the sake of the argument that the peptide
represents the conformationally flexible receptor and the water
molecule is the conformationally rigid drug molecule. The
anhydrous peptide is folded and is held together by an
intramolecular N-H..O = C (N..O = 2.97 Å) hydrogen bond (Fig. 6).
In the hydrated form a water molecule is inserted between the N
and O atoms and forms two intermolecular hydrogen bonds thereby
inducing a considerable conformational change (Fig. 7). In fact,
the N...O distance increased from 2.97 Å in the anhydrous form to
5.0 Å in the hydrated form. The extent of the conformational
difference is depicted in the superimposition shown in Fig. 8.

Let us envisage a possible scenario in which the water-free
intramolecularly hydrogen bonded peptide (A) is approached by a
water molecule. Then it is of importance to note that upon

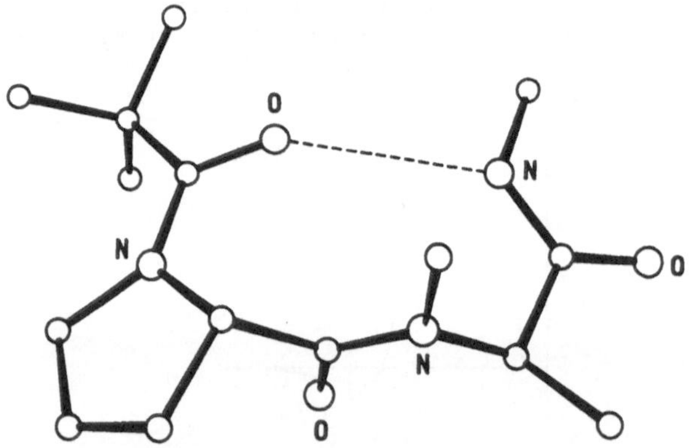

Fig. 6. Perspective drawing of anhydrous t-Bu-CO-L-Pro-Me-D-Ala-
NHMe (A). The hydrogen atoms are omitted for clarity.

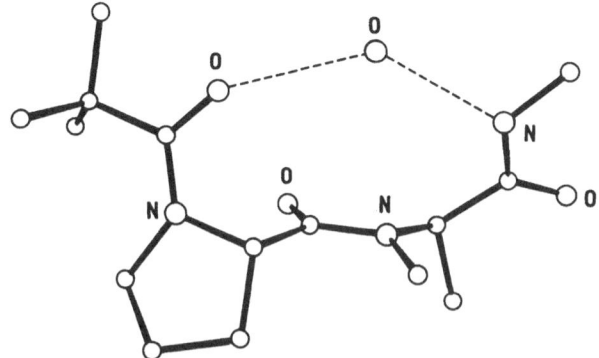

Fig. 7. Perspective drawing of hydrated t-Bu-CO-L-Pro-Me-D-Ala-NHMe (A.H$_2$O). The hydrogen atoms are omitted for clarity.

complex formation the intramolecular hydrogen bond is broken
followed by the formation of two intermolecular hydrogen bonds.
In other words, the net gain in stabilization energy with respect
to the hydrogen bonds is one intermolecular hydrogen bond.

$$E_{net} = (E_{NH..O_w})_{A.H_2O} + (E_{O_wH..O=})_{A.H_2O} - (E_{NH..O=})_A$$

$$E_{net} \approx (E_{O_wH..O=})_{A.H_2O} \approx 5 - 6 \text{ Kcal/mole}$$

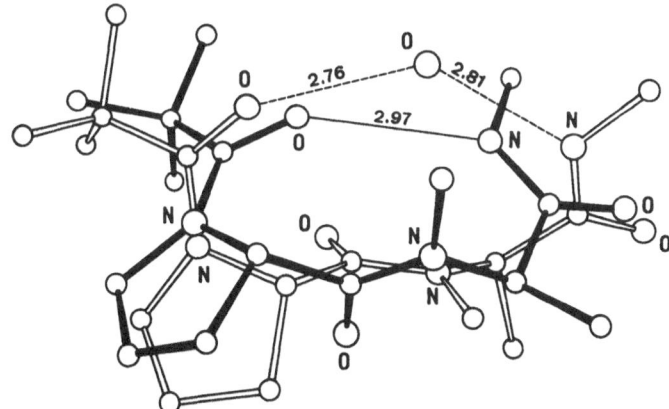

Fig. 8. Superimposition of anhydrous and hydrated t-Bu-CO-L-Pro-Me-D-Ala-NHMe.

203

That the net energy balance is not solely governed by the energy contributions of breaking and forming hydrogen bonds is suggested by semi-empirical quantum chemical computations (Diner et al., 1969). PCILO calculations based on the coordinates of the X-ray data of the hydrated peptide A show that the net stabilization energy E_{stab}

$$E_{stab} = E(A \cdot H_2O) - [E(H_2O) + E(A)] = 9.067 \text{ Kcal/mole}$$

In other words, PCILO calculations indicate that the resulting complex is some 9 Kcal/mole more stable than the reactants. The difference between E_{net} and E_{stab} of a few Kcal/mole may be accounted for by the additional energy gain due to the charge distribution reorganization and the consequences thereof in terms of eqs. 1 - 7 upon complex formation.

CONFORMATION ANALYSIS AND DRUG RESEARCH

As has been stated in a preceding section, conformation analysis yields in principle all energetically possible and impossible conformations in the absence of the receptor. In addition to this it is of interest to note that at best we have a rather sketchy idea of what a receptor looks like let alone some detailed geometrical information. Furthermore, as long as our ignorance concerning the conformation in the "fourth" aggregation state remains virtually complete we have to make do with the characterization of experimentally and theoretically determined conformations. If the objective is to deduce the pharmacophoric pattern that is responsible for activity the medicinal chemist will seek similarities and dissimilarities within a set of molecules supposedly acting on the same receptor. If the objective is to deduce the identity of the receptor, it might be a sobering thought that the saying (Pullman, 1976): "trying to guess the topography of the receptor from the study of the drug is like trying to guess the beauty of a lady from the picture of her husband" is still valid!

In what follows examples will be presented with mainly the first objective in mind. In other words, the primary task will be to deduce the pharmacophore from the conformational data of a given set of compounds. A pharmacophore can be defined as a set of atoms or chemical functions in a mutual orientation essential for recognition by and interaction with the receptor.

Let us assume that molecule A of Fig. 9 exhibits biological activity in a given test system and that molecule B is less active in the same test. Let it be further assumed that the

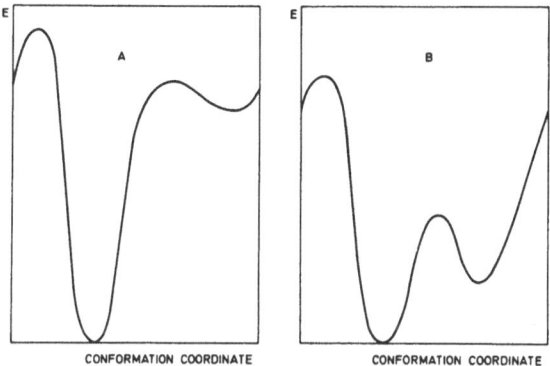

Fig. 9. Conformational profile of molecules A and B. The absolute energy minima of A and B are assumed to pertain to the biologically relevant conformation.

secondary minimum of A is energetically unacceptable i.e. that this minimum lies about 20 or more Kcal/mole higher than the absolute minimum which is therefore assumed to represent the biologically relevant conformation. From the conformational profile of molecules A and B one could hypothesize that the secondary conformational energy minimum of molecule B is biologically irrelevant as the common pharmacophoric pattern of A and B pertains to the absolute conformational minimum. Molecule B being less active than A may be rationalized by the fact that a certain mole fraction of B is in the biologically irrelevant conformation of the secondary energy minimum. Of course, other factors such as unfavourable lipophilicity differences between A and B may contribute or may even be the sole reason for the diminished activity of B.

In his study on the Baker triazines, Hopfinger (1980, 1981) proposed a biologically relevant conformation based on the reasoning described above and on the correlation with the biological activity of the test series of compounds.

An eloquent example of pharmacophoric pattern matching is furnished by the antimycotic agents miconazole and ketoconazole. From the classical structures presented in Fig. 10 it is not readily seen how both molecules are spatially related to one another. However, if the moieties known to be probably essential for antimycotic activity from previous qualitative structure-activity relationships, are superimposed by using the BMFIT (Best Molecular Fit Program, Nyburg, 1974) programme, a

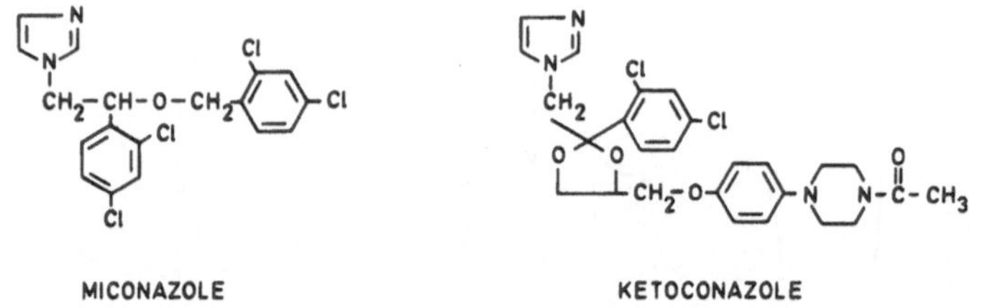

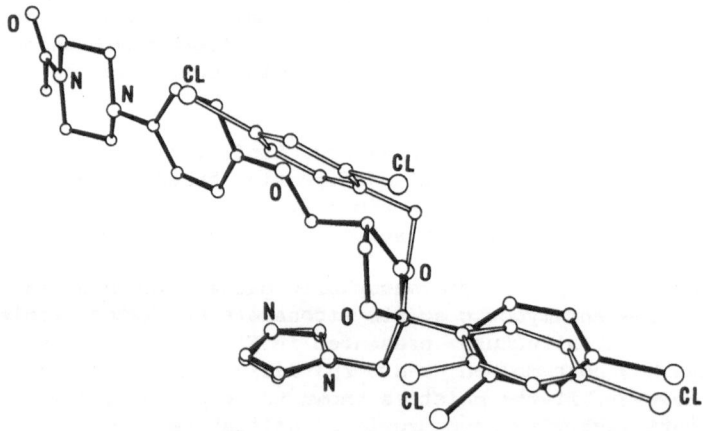

MICONAZOLE   KETOCONAZOLE

Fig. 10. Two-dimensional structure of miconazole and ketoconazole.

matching is obtained as shown in Fig. 11. It is seen that the
five-membered imidazole ring and the oxygen atoms of both
molecules in their crystal structure conformation (Blaton et al.,
1978; Peeters et al., 1979) almost perfectly match in space. The
planes of the 2,4-diCl substituted phenyl rings make an angle of
20°. Theoretical calculations, however, indicate that the phenyl
rings in both molecules have sufficient rotational freedom so
that both phenyl rings could become coplanar.

Knowledge of the pharmacophoric pattern assumed to be
responsible for a given biological response may then subsequently
be employed to devise new compounds possessing the pharmacophore
embedded in their structure. In the case of conformationally
flexible molecules a pharmacophoric pattern must be chosen from a
multitude of different conformations. The latter are usually
obtained from quantum chemical or empirical force field
calculations (Tollenaere, 1981).

Fig. 11. Superimposition of miconazole and ketoconazole.

CONCLUSIONS

The explosive growth of three-dimensional information on drug molecules during the last decade opens new avenues for the medicinal chemist. The concerted approach to drug design using theoretical and experimental methods for the determination of the three-dimensional features of different compounds leads to a better understanding of the factors involved in the pharmacological activity. Correlations between structure and activity, if any are possible, can then be used to identify stereochemical parameters which may form a basis for the design of new drugs. Although three-dimensional aspects have been heavily stressed in this contribution, it goes without saying that the medicinal chemist still should make changes in substituents attached to the pharmacophoric framework in order to maximize the factors governing the ability of the drug to reach the receptor site.

Acknowledgment. The author wishes to thank Mr. H. Moereels and Mrs. L. Raymaekers for their help in the preparation of the manuscript. Part of this work was supported by a grant of IWONL (Instituut tot Aanmoediging van het Wetenschappelijk Onderzoek in de Nijverheid en Landbouw).

REFERENCES

Albers-Schonberg, G., Arison, B.H., Chabala, J.C., Douglas, A.W., Eskola, P., Fisher, M.H., Lusi, A., Mrozik, H., Smith, J.L. and Tolman, R.L. (1981). Avermectins. Structure Determination. J. Am. Chem. Soc., 103, 4216-4221.

Aubry, A., Vitoux, B., Boussard, G. and Marraud, M. (1981). N-Methyl Peptides. IV. Water and ß-Turn in Peptides. Int. J. Peptide Protein Res., 18, 195-202.

Battershell, C., Malhotra, D. and Hopfinger, A.J. (1981). Inhibition of Dihydrofolate Reductase: Structure-Activity Correlations of Quinazolines Based upon Molecular Shape Analysis. J. Med. Chem., 24, 812-818.

Blaton, N.M., Peeters, O.M. and De Ranter, C.J. (1978). The Crystal and Molecular Structure of Trans-Tetrakis (miconazole) Cobalt (II) Nitrate, $(C_{18}H_{14}Cl_4N_2O)_4 Co(NO_3)_2$. Acta Cryst., B34, 1854-1857.

Chabala, J.C., Mrozik, H., Tolman, R.L., Eskola, P., Lusi, A., Peterson, L.H., Woods, M.F., Fisher, M., Campbell, W.C., Egerton, J.R. and Ostlind, D.A. (1980). Ivermectin, a New Broad-Spectrum Antiparasitic Agent. J. Med. Chem., 23, 1134-1136.

Cramer, R. (1980). A QSAR Success Story. Chemtech. 744-747.

Diner, S., Malrieu, J.P., Jordan, F. and Gilbert, M. (1969). Localized Bond Orbitals and the Correlation Problem. III. Energy up to the Third Order in the Zero-Differential Overlap Approximation. Application to σ-Electron Systems. Theor. Chim. Acta, 15, 100-110.

Hansch, C. and Fujita, T. (1964). ρ-σ-π Analysis. A Method for the Correlation of Biological Activity and Chemical Structure. J. Am. Chem. Soc., 86, 1616-1626.

Hansch, C. and Leo, A. (1979). Substituent Constants for Correlation Analysis in Chemistry and Biology. Wiley, New York.

Hopfinger, A.J. (1980). A QSAR Investigation of Dihydrofolate Reductase Inhibition by Baker Triazines Based upon Molecular Shape Analysis. J. Am. Chem. Soc., 102, 7196-7206.

Hopfinger, A.J. (1981). A General QSAR for Dihydrofolate Reductase Inhibition by 2,4-Diaminotriazines Based upon Molecular Shape Analysis. Arch. Biochem. Biophys., 206, 153-163.

Hopfinger, A.J. (1982). Ames Test and Antitumor Activity of 1-(X-Phenyl)-3,3-Dialkyltriazenes. Mol. Pharmacol., 21, 187-195.

Kollman, P.A. and Allen, L.C. (1972). The Theory of the Hydrogen Bond. Chem. Rev., 72, 283-303.

Martin, Y. (1981). A Practitioner's Perspective of the Role of Quantitative Structure-Activity Analysis in Medicinal Chemistry. J. Med. Chem., 24, 230-237.

McGuire, R.F., Momamy, F.A. and Scheraga, H.A. (1972). Energy Parameters in Polypeptides. V. An Empirical Hydrogen Bond Potential Function Based on Molecular Orbital Calculations. J. Phys. Chem., 76, 375-393.

Nyburg, S.C. (1974). Some Uses of a Best Molecular Fit Routine. Acta Cryst. B30, 251-253.

Pullman, B. (1976). Orbitals, Conformation and Biological Activity. Methods of Computation. Trends in Biochemical Sciences, N130-N131.

Peeters, O.M., Blaton, N.M. and De Ranter, C.J. (1979). Cis-1-Acetyl-4-(4-{[2-(2,4-dichlorophenyl)-2-(1H-1-imidazolylmethyl)-1,3-dioxolan-4-yl]methoxy} phenyl)piperazine: Ketoconazole. A Crystal Structure with Disorder. Acta Cryst., B35, 2461-2464.

Springer, J.P., Arison, B.H., Hirshfield, J.M. and Hoogsteen, K. (1981). The Absolute Stereochemistry and Conformation of Avermectin B_{2a} Aglycon and Avermectin B_{1a}. J. Am. Chem. Soc., 103, 4221-4224.

Stuper, A.J., Dyott, T.M. and Zander, G.S. (1979). Conformational Analysis: A Module in a Program for the Design of Biologically Active Compounds. In Computer-Assisted Drug Design (eds. E.C. Olson and R.E. Christoffersen). American Chemical Society Symposium Series 112.

Tollenaere, J.P. (1973). Structure-Activity Relationships of Three Groups of Uncouplers of Oxidative Phosphorylation: Salicylanilides, 2-Trifluoromethylbenzimidazoles, and Phenols. J. Med. Chem., 16, 791-796.

Tollenaere, J.P., Moereels, H. and Van den Bossche, H. (1976). Comparison of the Structure-Activity Relationships of Substituted Phenols as Uncouplers of Oxidative Phosphorylation in Rat Liver and Ascaris Muscle Mitochondria. In Biochemistry of Parasites and Host-Parasite Relationships. (ed. H. Van den Bossche). Elsevier/North-Holland Biomedical Press, Amsterdam.

Tollenaere, J.P., Moereels, H. and Raymaekers, L.A. (1979). Atlas of the Three-Dimensional Structure of Drugs. Elsevier/North-Holland Biomedical Press, Amsterdam.

Tollenaere, J.P., Moereels, H. and Raymaekers, L.A. (1980). Structural Aspects of the Structure-Activity Relationships of Neuroleptics: Principles and Methods. In Drug Design, Vol. X (ed. E.J. Ariëns). Academic Press, New York.

Tollenaere, J.P. (1981). Conformational Analysis in Medicinal Chemistry. Trends in Pharmacological Sciences, 2, 273-275.

Targeting of drugs with liposomes

G Gregoriadis

Division of Clinical Sciences, Clinical Research Centre,
Watford Road, Harrow, Middlesex, HA1 3UJ, UK

Introduction

At least two options are open to us in pursuing optimal drug
action (Gregoriadis, 1981a). In the first, creation of
specialised molecules, a therapeutically profitable target-drug
relationship is usually far from ideal and undesirable side
effects are almost always present. In the second, drug molecules
that are not necessarily target specific are transported by a
carrier to the area of action and subsequently allowed to perform
their task. Transport by the carrier should be effected in
isolation from the biological space existing between the site of
application and the site of action as this would be useful in
cases where drugs are either prone to premature excretion and
inactivation or detrimental to the non-target space in the host.
The carrier itself should be non-toxic, biodegradable and of the
appropriate shape and size so as to enable accommodation of a
wide variety of therapeutic agents. It should preferably ignore
or be ignored by irrelevant (normal) areas and have a pronounced
affinity for, and access to the target site within which there
should be a mechanism for the release of agents from the carrier.
The latter, having accomplished its function, should then be
disposed of.

Intensive work during the last decade (Gregoriadis, et al.,
1982a) suggests that liposomes as a carrier candidate can fulfil
many of these requirements. Liposomes are formed when water-
insoluble polar lipids (namely phospholipids) are confronted with
water. The highly ordered assemblages that emerge persist in the
presence of excess water and, being associated with unfavourable
entropy, are finally arranged in a system of concentric closed
membranes. Upon sonication, these multilamellar liposomes can
break up to form smaller unilamellar structures. Before
closed structures form, there is unrestricted entry of water and

solutes (eg. drugs) in between the planes of polar head groups.
Thus, water soluble substances can be entrapped in the aqueous
compartments provided that such substances do not interfere with
liposome formation and that their size is compatible with the
dimensions of the aqueous space between the planes of the
hydrophilic head groups (about 7.5 nm in width) or of the space
of unilamellar liposomes (about 8.5 nm in diameter). In
multilamellar liposomes there is a much larger aqueous core
(about 0.15 μm). Alternatively, lipid soluble substances can be
accommodated in the lipid phase of liposomes. Further
developments in liposome technology have led to the preparation
of vesicles of a variety of sizes and properties that can be
tailored to specific needs (Leserman and Barbet, 1982;
Gregoriadis, 1983).

Behaviour of liposomes in vivo

Injected liposomes, depending on their route of administration

and structural characteristics (eg. stability, size, surface
charge, lipid composition), transport drugs into various cell
types in the liver, spleen, lungs and lymph nodes, mostly by
endocytosis. In addition, conditions have been established that
favour introduction of liposomal agents into distinct
intracellular sites in vitro (Poste 1980; Gregoriadis 1981a).
Recently there have been concerted attempts to alter the
structure and composition of liposomes so as to design vesicles
that exhibit well-defined behaviour in a given environment. For
instance, high-density lipoproteins in the blood remove
phospholipid molecules from liposomes (Scherphof et al., 1978;
Chobanian et al., 1979) to render them leaky (Kirby and
Gregoriadis, 1981) to entrapped drugs. By adjusting the
cholesterol content of the bilayers, lipoprotein action can be
controlled so as to achieve optimum rates of drug leakage from
circulating liposomes or, when drugs must be carried in bulk
(without loss through leakage) to the target, to abolish leakage
altogether (Kirby et al., 1980a,b; Kirby and Gregoriadis 1980).
The scope of such control is further expanded by the appropriate
choice of the phospholipid component which will determine the
half-life of the carrier in the circulation (Gregoriadis and
Senior, 1980; Senior and Gregoriadis, 1982). Judicious
manipulation of these and other liposomal characteristics can,
therefore, provide a wide range of options in controlled drug
release or transport via stable liposomes (Gregoriadis et al.,
1982a). In another case of milieu exploitation advantage is taken
of subtle differences in pH values between certain tumours or
inflamed tissues and their normal surroundings. Thus, pH-sensitive molecules incorporated into drug-carrying liposomes could, at
a narrow pH range, destabilise the bilayers and induce drug
leakage near areas in need of treatment (Yatvin et al., 1980).

Structural changes can also optimise the action of liposomal drugs administered locally. For instance, certain sugar or aminosugar derivatives incorporated onto the surface of liposomes mediate the latter's long-term (up to several days) retention by cells to which they bind at the site of injection (Mauk et al., 1980). A different approach towards improving liposomal drug action is the design of liposomes that work best in environments amenable to modification. An interesting example is liposomes made of suitable mixtures of phospholipids that "melt" at temperatures slightly above 37°C to release drug contents. Heated tumours in animals injected with temperature-sensitive liposomes were thus shown to accumulate more drug that unheated ones (Weinstein et al., 1979).

As the range of cell types (mostly phagocytes) with which conventional liposomes associate in vivo is rather limited, efforts have been made to widen their spectrum of localisation (Gregoriadis et al., 1982a). Anti-tumour cell antibodies incorporated onto the surface of drug-containing liposomes were found to mediate uptake of the latter by the tumour cells in vitro (Gregoriadis and Neerunjun 1975; Leserman et al., 1980; Heath et al., 1980; Huang et al., 1980). Targeting in tumour- bearing animals with similar antibody-bearing liposomes was not, however, as successful (Gregoriadis and Neerunjun, 1975). That liposomes could target in vivo was, nonetheless, demonstrated by coating them with desialylated fetuin (Gregoriadis and Neerunjun, 1975) which mediated liposome uptake by the hepatic parenchymal cells bearing the appropriate receptor. There has been further progress in targeting liposomes with antibodies, especially with regard to techniques of linking these to the liposomal surface (Gregoriadis et al., 1982a). Of particular interest is the use of monoclonal antibodies, which have improved the binding of liposomes to cells in vitro (Leserman et al., 1980; Huang et al., 1980).

Applications in medicine

Work in animals has significantly advanced the prospect of using liposomes in medicine. Initially, the observation that liposomes are lysosomotropic raised hopes for their suitability in enzyme therapy of lysosomal storage diseases. After studies with model storage conditions, the approach was tested in patients with Gaucher's disease type I. In a 5-year period of treatment one of the patients with hepatomegaly received over 60 intravenous injections of liposome-entrapped human glucocerebroside: β-glucosidase. Physical examination, as well as serial ultrasound scans of the liver in one case, indicates that general health and size of the liver have, at the very least, remained unchanged through the years. To my knowledge this is the only study of long-term exposure of man to liposomes and has revealed through haematological and other tests that multilamellar liposomes composed of egg phosphatidylcholine, cholesterol, and phosphatidic acid have no obvious untoward effects (Gregoriadis, et al., (1982b).

213

Additional conditions involving the reticuloendothelial system and thus amenable to treatment with liposomal drugs are parasitic diseases, in which microbes reside within the fixed macrophages. Such diseases are of particular concern because of the very great number of people affected and the ineffectiveness and/or toxicity of available antimicrobial agents. Several workers (Alving et al., 1978; Black et al., 1977; New et al., 1978) have now shown that experimental visceral and cutaneous leishmaniasis in animals can be treated successfully with small amounts of liposome-entrapped antimonial drugs. Another important group of reticuloendothelial-system diseases includes those in which metals accumulate intracellularly. However, chelators designed to relieve cells from excess metal cross membranes rather poorly. Results from animals loaded with plutonium, mercury, colloidal gold, or iron and injected with chelator-containing liposomes have again demonstrated the therapeutic value of the system (Rahman, 1980).

Several groups have investigated the potential of liposomes as a drug delivery system in the treatment of cancer (Gregoriadis, 1981a). However, actual transport of drugs to tumour cells has not as yet been proven and encouraging results with ascites and solid tumours in rodents treated with liposomal phase-specific drugs are presently attributed to the slow release of drugs from the circulating carrier (Gregoriadis, 1981). An alternative way to use liposomes in cancer therapy employs their natural affinity for macrophages. For instance, liposomes contain ing macrophage activation factors will convert resting macrophages to an activated state with increased ability to kill tumours in vitro and in vivo and without significant toxicity to normal tissues (Poste et al., 1979; Fiddler, 1980). Treatment of cancer by the administration of liposomal drugs through routes other than the intravenous has also been proposed. Interesting examples are intratracheal instillation for the treatment of lung cancer (McCullough and Juliano, 1979) and subcutaneous injection for the imaging and treatment of metastases in lymph nodes draining the injected tissue (Segal et al., 1975; Osborne et al., 1979).

Other potential applications of interest include intragast-ric and intraarticular treatment. With regard to the former, various reports (Dapergolas and Gregoriadis, 1976; Ryman et al., 1978) on the glucose lowering effect of liposomal insulin in diabetic, and a single study (Hemker et al., 1980) in which oral administration of liposomal factor VIII into a patient with haemophilia A led to therapeutic levels of the factor in the blood, raised hoped for the oral treatment of the two diseases. However, reduced liposomal stability in the gut and poor absorption of both insulin (Dapergolas and Gregoriadis, 1976) and factor VIII (Hemker et al, 1980) have made apparent the need for radical modifications of the carrier (Gregoriadis, 1980).

214

Finally, promotion of humoral and cell-mediated immune responses to entrapped antigens by liposomes, is probably one of the more promising aspects of this carrier system in terms of early clinical application (Gregoriadis, 1981b). Several bacterial and viral antigens of relevance to human diseases have been entrapped in liposomes which were shown to act as a powerful immunological adjuvant (Gregoriadis, 1981b). In contrast to other adjuvants that are either toxic or ineffective, liposomes are generally innocuous and can be designed on a rational basis to produce safe and efficient vaccines for human and animal immunization programs.

Recent studies in this laboratory (Gregoriadis and Manesis, 1980) indicate that liposomes hold promise as an adjuvant for a hepatitis B vaccine. HB_sAg can readily be incorporated into multilamellar liposomes and immunization of guinea pigs with liposomal HB_sAg as such or in mixture with killed B. pertussis or saponin produces earlier conversion rates and higher antibody responses (750 times at the end of several weeks) than with the free antigen alone or in association with the two other adjuvants. Interestingly, delayed hypersensitivity tests show that the immune response is cell-mediated as well. This should be an advantage since there is strong evidence that cell-mediated immunity plays a major role in the protection against most viral infections. Encouraging results have also been obtained (Gregoriadis and Manesis, 1980) in inbred mice where a single injection of the liposomal HB_sAg produced plateau antibody values lasting for at least 130 days. From comparative studies, it appears that liposomal HB_sAg can be more effective than HB_sAg aministered with a variety of other adjuvants including alum oxide, muramyl dipeptide, and complete Freund's adjuvant. It should be noted that although in a recent clinical trial (Szmuness et al., 1980) vaccination with HB_sAg the use of alum as an adjuvant has proved successful, the tendency of antibody titers to decline several months after the first injection may affect long-term protection from the disease. Furthermore, the individuals in this trials (Szmuness et al., 1980) were injected three times, a practice with obvious socioeconomic disadvantages. It remains to be seen whether, with smaller amounts of antigen and fewer injections, liposomes can prolong further HB_sAg antibody titers in humans. Other important features of liposomes as immunologic adjuvants also merit discussion. For instance, among a variety of synthetic adjuvants, liposomes are unique in their flexibility in composition and structure. This enables us to control their behaviour in vivo so as to satisfy particular needs. As already discussed, manipulation of size, surface charge, and phospholipid composition can influence the rate of clearance of liposomes from the injected site or from the blood and their uptake by tissues. Such modifications, in conjunction with the control of entrapped antigen diffusion from liposomes in situ (eg. through the adjustment of their cholesterol content; Kirby et al, 1980a), may lead to patterns of antigen distribution

215

and fate compatible with augmented immunogenicity and may help in producing "single shot" vaccines.

Two aspects of liposomes that concern pharmaceutical industries are stability under storage and toxicity. Developments in this and other laboratories (Gregoriadis et al., 1982a) suggest that liposomes can be made to preserve their structural integrity for prolonged periods of time and, at the same time, retain entrapped agents quantitatively. With some of the agents liposomal preparations can even be lyophilized. There is also evidence that liposomes, when of appropriate lipid composition, are not toxic and do not form antibodies against their lipid constituents. However, the possibility remains that liposome-associated antigens or synergistically acting adjuvants can induce antibody response to the liposomal lipids. There is growing optimism that such problems, if present, can be circumvented.

References

Alving, C.R., Steck, E.A., Chapman, Jr, W.L., Waits, V.B., Hendricks, L.D., Swartz, Jr., G.M.., Hanson, W.L. (1978). Therapy of leishmaniasis: superior efficacies of liposome encapsulated drugs. Proc. Nat. Acad. Sci. USA, 75, 2959-63.

Black, C.D.V., Watson, C.J., Ward, R.J. (1977). The use of pentostam liposomes in the chemotherapy of experimental leishmaniasis. Trans. Roy. Soc. Trop. Med. Hyg. 71, 550-52.

Chobanian, J.V., Tall, A.R., Brecher, P.I. (1979). Interaction between unilamellar egg yolk lecithin vesicles and human high density lipoproteins. Biochemistry, 18, 180-87.

Dapergolas, G. and Gregoriadis, G. (1976) Hypoglycaemic effect of liposome-entrapped insulin administered intragastrically into rats. Lancet ii, 824-27.

Fidler, I.J. (1980). Therapy of spontaneous metastases by intravenous injection of liposomes containing lymphokines. Science, 108, 1469-71.

Gregoriadis, G., (1981). Liposomes: a role in vaccines?. Clin Immunol Newsl. 2, 33-36.

Gregoriadis, G., Manesis, E.K. (1980). Liposomes as immunological adjuvants for hepatitis B surface antigens. In: Liposomes and immunobiology (eds. B.H. Tom and H.R. Six). Elsevier/North Holland, New York, Amsterdam.

Gregoriadis, G. (1981a). Targeting of drugs: implications in medicine. The Lancet, 2, 241-247.

Gregoriadis, G., Senior, J. and Trouet, A. (eds.) (1982a). Targeting of drugs. Plenum, New York.

Gregoriadis, G. and Senior, J. (1980). The phospholipid components of small unilamellar liposome controls the rate of clearance of entrapped solutes from the circulation. FEBS Lett 119, 43-46.

Gregoriadis, G. (1983). Liposomes Technology. CRC Press Inc. Florida (In press).

Leserman, L.D. and Barbet, J. (eds.) (1982). Méthodologie des liposomes, Inserm, Paris.

Huang, A., Huang, L. and Kennel, S.J. (1980). Monoclonal antibody covalently coupled with fatty acid. J. Biol. Chem., 255, 8015-8018.

Kirby, C. and Gregoriadis, G. (1981). Plasma-induced release of solutes from small unilamellar liposomes is associated with pore formation in the bilayers. Biochem. J. 199, 251-254.

Kirby, C., Clark, J. and Gregoriadis, G. (1980a). Effect of the cholesterol content of small unilamellar liposomes on their stability in vivo and in vitro. Biochem. J. 186, 591-598.

Kirby, C., Clarke, J. and Gregoriadis, G. (1980b). Cholesterol content of small unilamellar liposomes controls phospholipid loss to high density lipoproteins in the presence of serum. FEBS Lett 111, 324-328.

Kirby, C. and Gregoriadis, G. (1980). The effect of the cholesterol content of small unilamellar liposomes on the fate of their lipid components in vivo. Life Sci, 27, 2223-2230.

Leserman, L.D., Barbet, J., Kourisky, F. and Weinstein, J.N. (1980). Targeting to cells of fluorescent liposomes covalently coupled with monoclonal antibody of protein A. Nature, 288, 602-604.

Mauk, M.R., Gamble, R.C. and Baldeschwieler, J.D. Targeting of lipid vesicles : specificity of carbohydrate receptor analogues for leucocytes in mice. Proc. Nat. Acad. Sci. USA 77, 4430-4434.

McCullough, H.N. and Juliano, R.L. (1979). Organ-selective action of an antitumour drug: pharmacologic studies of liposome-encapsulated β-cytosine arabinoside administered via the respiratory system of the rat. J. Nat. Cancer. Inst., 63, 727-731.

New, R.R.C., Chance, M.L., Thomas, S.C. and Peters, W. (1978). Antileishmanial activity of antimonial entrapped in liposomes. Nature, 272, 55-56.

Osborne, M.P., Richardson, V.J., Jehasingh, K. and Ryman, B.E. (1979). Radionuclide-labelled liposomes: a new lymph node imaging agent. J. Nucl. Med. Biol., 675-683.

Poste, G., Kirsh, R., Fogler, W.E. and Fidler, I.J. (1979). Activation of tumourcidal properties in mouse macrophages by lymphokines encapsulated in liposomes. Cancer Res., 39, 881-892.

Poste, G. (1980). The interaction of lipid vesicles (liposomes) with cultured cells and their use as carriers for drugs and macromolecules. In: Liposomes in biological systems. (eds. G. Gregoriadis and A.C. Allison) John Wiley and Sons. Chichester, New York

Rahman, Y.E. (1980). Liposomes and chelating agents. In: Liposomes in biological systems. (eds. G. Gregoriadis, and A.C. Allison. John Wiley and Sons. Chichester, New York.

Ryman, B.E., Jewkes, R.F. and Jegsingh, K. (1978) Potential applications of liposomes to therapy. Ann NY Acad Sci, 308, 281-307.

Gregoriadis, G., Weereratne, H., Blair, H. and Bull, G.M. (1982b) Liposomes in Gaucher's disease type I : use in therapy and the creation of an animal model. In: Gaucher's disease. The most prevalent Jewish genetic disease (ed. R.J. Desnick) Alan L. Liss, New York.

Gregoriadis, G. and Neerunjun, E.D., (1975). Homing of liposomes to target cells. Biochem. Biophys. Res. Comm. 65, 537-44.

Heath, T.D., Fraley, R.T. and Papahadjopoulos, D. (1980). Antibody targeting of liposomes: cell specificity obtained by conjugation of F(ab') to vesicle surface. Science, 210, 539-41.

Hemker, HJ.C., Muller, A.D., Hermans, W. Th. and Swaal, R.F.A. (1980). Oral treatment of haemophilia A by gastrointestinal absorption of factor VIII entrapped in liposomes. Lancet, i, 70-71.

Scherphof, G., Roerdink, F., Waite, M. and Parks, J. (1978). Disintegration of phosphatidylcholine liposomes in plasma as a result of interaction with high-density lipoproteins. Biochim. Biophys. Acta. 542, 296-307.

Segal, A.W., Gregoriadis, G. and Black, C.D.V. (1975). Liposomes as vehicles for the local release of drugs. Clin. Sci. Mol. Med., 49, 99-106.

Senior, J. and Gregoriadis, G. (1982). Stability of small unilamellar liposomes in serum and clearance from the circulation :
the effect of the phospholipid and cholesterol components. Life
Sci. 30, 2123-2136.

Szmuness, S., Stevens, C.E., Harley, E.J., Zang, E.A., Eleszko,
W.R., Williams, D.C., Sadovsky, R., Morrison, J.M. and Kellner,
A. (1980). Hepatitis B vaccine. Demonstration of efficiency in a
controlled clinical trial in a high risk population in the USA.
N. Engl. J. Med. 303, 833-841.

Weinstein, J.N., Magin R.L., Yatvin, M.B. and Saharko, D.S.
(1979). Liposomes and local hyperthermia; delivery of
methotrexate to heated tumours. Science, 204, 188-91.

Yatvin, M.B., Kreutz, W., Horwitz, B.A. and Shinitzky, M. (1980).
pH-sensitive liposomes : Possible clinical implications.
Science, 210, 1353-55.

Index

225

Levamisole (continued)
  resistance to, 117
  structure, 111
Lewis lung carcinoma system,
    135
Lipophilicity, 161, 193, 205
  effects of, 185
Liposomes, 211
  and carrier transport, 211
  multilamellar, 211
  unilamellar, 211
  behaviour in vivo, 212
  route of administration, 212
  structural characteristics,
    212
  cholesterol content of, 212
  phospholipid content of, 212
  pH sensitive molecules and,
    212
  drug-carrying, 212
  structural changes of, 212
  and anti-tumour cell anti-
      bodies, 213
  antibody bearing, 213
  and desialytated fetuin, 213
  and monoclonal antibodies,
    213
  medical applications of, 213
  and parasitic disease, 213
  and Gaucher's disease, 213
  and leishmaniasis, 213
  and metal accumulation, 214
  and treatment of cancer, 214
  affinity for macrophages, 214
  macrophage activation factors
      of, 214
  intratracheal instillation
      of, 214
  subcutaneous injection of,
    214
  intragastric treatment with,
    214
  intraarticular treatment
      with, 214
  treatment of diabetes with,
    214
  and entrapped antigens, 214
  as adjuvants, 215
  Hb$_s$Ag, 215
  and alum oxide, 215
  and muramyl dipeptide, 215

Liposomes (continued)
  and Freund's adjuvant, 215
  and Hepatitis B vaccine, 215
  stability of, 215
  toxicity of, 215
  lyophilization of, 216
  and Leishmania, 94
  and Plasmodium, 93, 94, 95
  containing sodium
      stibogluconate, 94
  containing glycolipids, 94
  cholesterol-rich, 95
Location of infection, 151
London Interactions, 201
LY127935, see Moxalactam
Lysosomal storage disease, 212

Macaca mulatta, 110
Macrolide
  resistance, 80
Macrophages, 213
  and liposomes, 214
Matrix algebra, 180, 182
Mebendazole, 105
  and onchocerciasis, 106
  combination with levamisole,
    106
  inhibition constant of, 107
  pharmacokinetic behaviour,
    106, 107
  primary site of action, 108
  structure, 111
Mecillinam, 54, 55
Mefloquin, 87
Melarsoprol, 86
  reactive encephalopathy with,
    86
Mel B, see Melarsoprol
Melphalan, 165
Membrane Active Antimicrobial
      Agents, 25
Membrane hyperpolarization, 115
Metastasis, 135, 136, 137, 138
Methicillin, 50, 51
6-Methoxy-8-aminoquinoline, see
      Primaquine
2'-0-methyladenosine, 74
Methyl-2-benzimidazole
      carbamate, 108
Methyridine, 109
  structure, 111

227